Table of Contents

Table of Contents 1
Free Gift 8
Introduction 9
Dash Diet Slow Cooker Breakfast Recipes 10
    Delicious Apple Granola Breakfast 10
    Delicious Banana and Coconut Oatmeal 10
    Carrot and Zucchini Oatmeal 11
    Coconut Quinoa Mix 11
    Simple Banana Bread 12
    Greek Dash Casserole 12
    Easy Breakfast Casserole 13
    Mexican Dash Diet Eggs 13
    Simple Apple Oatmeal 14
    Easy Quinoa and Oats 14
    Easy Pumpkin Oatmeal 15
    Raspberry Oatmeal 15
    Delicious Frittata 16
    Spinach Frittata 16
    Breakfast Veggie Omelet 17
    Scrambled Eggs 17
    Apple and Raisins Oatmeal 18
    Delicious Peanut Butter Oats 18
    Orange and Strawberry Breakfast Mix 19
    Delicious Omelet 19
    Fruits and Cereals Mix 20
    Breakfast Berries Compote 20
    Apples and Dates Oatmeal 21
    Scrambled Eggs and Veggies 21
    Mexican Casserole 22
    Shrimp Frittata 22
    Tofu Scramble 23
    Squash and Apples Breakfast Mix 23
    Corn Pudding 24
    Sweet Potatoes Mix 24
    Almond and Cherries Oats 25
    Cranberry Toast 25
    Easy Burrito Bowls 26
    Spiced Coconut Oats 26
    Easy Carrot Oatmeal 27
    Simple Blueberries Oatmeal 27
    Tofu and Veggies Frittata 28

Chia Pudding...28
Breakfast Potatoes..29
Breakfast Nuts and Squash Bowls...29
Leeks, Kale and Sweet Potato Mix..30
Egg Casserole...30
Maple Apples...31
Apples and Sauce...31
Sweet Potato and Sausage Pie..32
Pumpkin Butter..32
Pineapple and Carrot Mix..33
Spinach Pie..33
Creamy Veggie Omelet..34
Salmon Omelet..34
Chicken Omelet...35

Dash Diet Slow Cooker Main Dish Recipes 36
Chicken Tacos..36
Quinoa Casserole...36
Quinoa Curry...37
Delicious Black Bean Chili...37
Chicken and Veggies..38
Succulent Pork Roast...38
Turkey Chili...39
Easy Pulled Chicken..39
Mediterranean Chicken...40
Delicious Veggie Soup...40
Chicken and Rice Soup..41
Delicious Black Bean Soup..41
Beet Soup...42
Delicious Tomato Cream...42
Rich Lentils Soup...43
Broccoli and Cauliflower Soup..43
Butternut Squash Cream...44
Chickpeas Mix...44
Navy Beans Stew..45
Potatoes Stew...45
Easy Navy Beans Soup..46
Black Beans and Mango Mix...46
Spinach Soup...47
Asian Salmon..47
Seafood Stew..48
Slow Cooked Tuna...48
Herbed Salmon...49
Coconut Clams..49

Creamy Seafood and Veggies Soup 50
Seafood Gumbo 50
Lemon and Spinach Trout 51
Mexican Chicken 51
Chicken Breast Stew 52
Turkey Breast and Sweet Potato Mix 52
Italian Chicken.. 53
Chicken Breast and Cinnamon Veggie Mix 53
Mexican Pork Mix 54
Maple Pork Tenderloin 54
Pork and Cabbage Stew 55
Greek Pork 55
Roast and Veggies 56
Pork Roast Soup 56
Coconut Salmon Soup 57
Ground Pork and Veggies Soup 57
Greek Cod Mix 58
Creamy Fish Curry 58
Hot Mackerel 59
Mussels Mix 59
Turkey Wings and Veggies 60
Citrus Turkey Mix... 60

Dash Diet Slow Cooker Side Dish Recipes 61
Broccoli Mix 61
Tasty Bean Side Dish 61
Easy Green Beans 62
Creamy Corn.. 62
Classic Peas and Carrots 63
Mushroom Pilaf.. 63
Butternut Mix... 64
Sausage Side Dish 64
Easy Potatoes Mix 65
Black-Eyed Peas Mix.. 65
Green Beans and Corn Mix 66
Spiced Carrots.. 66
Squash and Grains Mix 67
Mushroom Mix... 67
Spinach and Rice 68
Creamy Mushrooms Mix 68
Ginger Beets 69
Artichokes Mix 69
Asparagus Mix 70
Black Bean and Corn Mix... 70

Celery Mix 71
Kale Side Dish 71
Spicy Eggplant 72
Corn Salad 72
Spiced Cabbage 73
Spinach and Beans Mix 73
Sage Sweet Potatoes 74
Garlicky Potato Mash 74
Chickpeas Side Dish 75
Warm Eggplant Salad 75
Garlic and Rosemary Potato Mix 76
Apple Brussels Sprouts 76
Italian Beans Mix 77
Tomatoes, Okra and Zucchini Mix 77
Easy Cabbage 78
Acorn Squash Mix 78
Italian Zucchini and Squash 79
Coconut Broccoli 79
Asian Green Beans 80
Cauliflower Rice and Mushrooms 80
Cranberries, Cauliflower and Mushroom Mix 81
Creamy Cauliflower Rice 81
Creamy and Cheesy Spinach 82
Dill Cauliflower Mash 82
Baby Spinach and Avocado Mix 83
Simple Parsnips Mix 83
Basil and Oregano Mushrooms 84
Minty Okra 84
Cabbage, Radish and Carrot Mix 85
Simple Swiss Chard Mix 85
Dash Diet Slow Cooker Snack and Appetizer Recipes 86
Eggplant Salsa 86
Artichoke and Beans Spread 86
Stuffed White Mushrooms 87
Italian Tomato Appetizer 87
Sweet Pineapple Snack 88
Chickpeas Hummus 88
Asparagus Snack 89
Shrimp and Beans Appetizer Salad 89
Pepper and Chickpeas Dip 90
White Bean Spread 90
Minty Spinach Dip 91
Turnips and Cauliflower Spread 91

Italian Veggie Dip	92
Cajun Peas Spread	92
Cashew Spread	93
Coconut Spinach Dip	93
Black Bean Salsa	94
Chili Coconut Corn Spread	94
Artichoke and Spinach Dip	95
Mushroom and Bell Pepper Dip	95
Warm French Veggie Salad	96
Bulgur and Beans Salad	96
Pineapple Chicken Wings	97
Spiced Pecans Snack	97
Easy Pork Party Meatballs	98
Pork Rolls	98
Tomato Salsa	99
White Fish Sticks	99
Tomato Shrimp Salad	100
Stuffed Chicken	100
Italian Nuts Mix	101
Dill Walnuts and Seeds Mix	101
Tomato Dip	102
Zucchini Dip	102
Easy Zucchini Rolls	103
Jumbo Shrimp Appetizer	103
Salmon Appetizer Salad	104
Beet and Celery Spread	104
Clams Salad	105
Creamy Endive Salad	105
Chili Cauliflower Dip	106
Cranberries, Apple and Onion Salad	106
Sausage Meatballs and Apricot Sauce	107
Sriracha Chicken Dip	107
Shrimp Cocktail	108
Cod Salsa	108
Salmon and Carrots Appetizer Salad	109
Italian Shrimp Salad	109
Salmon and Scallions Salad	110
Salmon Bites and Lemon Dressing	110
Dash Diet Slow Cooker Dessert Recipes	**111**
Easy Carrot and Pineapple Cake	111
Coconut Green Tea Cream	111
Sweet Coconut Figs	112
Chocolate and Vanilla Cream	112

Cinnamon Tomato Mix	113
Tomato Pie	113
Berries and Orange Sauce	114
Mango and Orange Sauce	114
Sweet Minty Grapefruit Mix	115
Plums Stew	115
Cinnamon Apples	116
Cocoa Cake	116
Blueberry Pie	117
Coconut Peach Cobbler	117
Poached Strawberries	118
Poached Bananas	118
Orange and Pecans Cake	119
Poached Pears	119
Pumpkin Pie	120
Lemon Cream	120
Minty Rhubarb Dip	121
Cherry Jam	121
Cinnamon Rice Pudding	122
Almond Chocolate Bars	122
Pineapple Pudding	123
Delicious Apple Mix	123
Avocado Pudding	124
Chia Pudding	124
Grapefruit Compote	125
Dark Cherry and Cocoa Compote	125
Citrus Apples and Pears Mix	126
Pears Cake	126
Cocoa Pudding	127
Raspberry Energy Bars	127
Berries Cream	128
Blackberries and Cocoa Pudding	128
Peach Compote	129
Zucchini Cake	129
Grapes Pudding	130
Apricot Cream	130
Poached Apples	131
Stewed Cardamom Pears	131
Maple Grapes Compote	132
Brown Rice Pudding	132
Berry Cobbler	133
Pumpkin Apple Dip	133
Apple Dip	134

 Cranberry Dip.. 134
 Sweet Mango Dip... 135
 Plum Dip 135
Conclusion 136
Recipe Index... 137

Free Gift

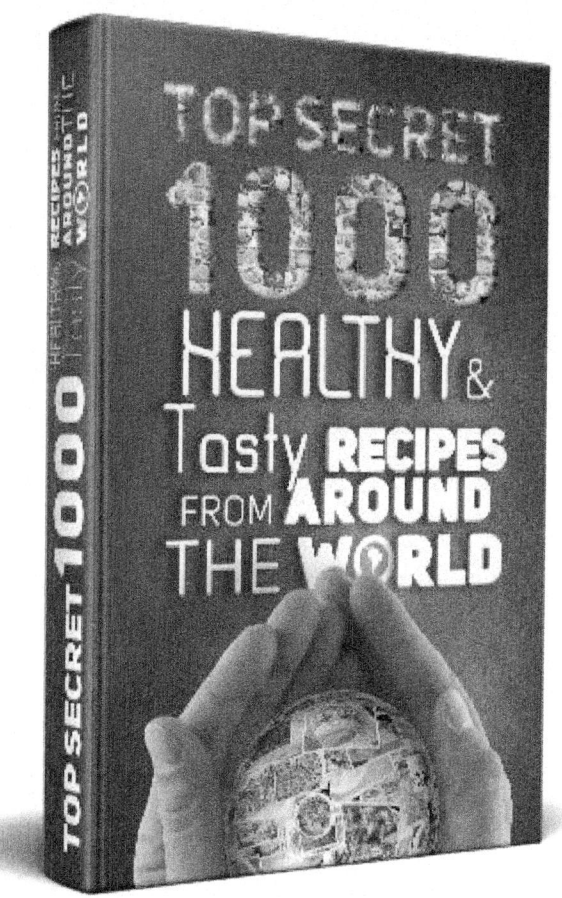

Up to 1000 delicious and healthy recipes from cooking traditions all around the world.

Please follow this link to get instant access to your Free Cookbook:
http://bookretailseller.pro/

Introduction

What is the Dash diet and why are so many people interested in following it these days? That's exactly what we want you to discover today! We are sure that once you find out everything there is to know about the Dash diet you will decide to make it your lifestyle.

The Dash diet stands for Dietary Approaches to Stop Hypertension. It's a healthy lifestyle that was developed in order to prevent high blood pressure, which is one important factor in heart disease.
Also, the Dash diet is a simple and easy way to lose some extra weight and to become a happier and healthier person.

The Dash diet is based on reducing the amount of sodium you consume each day and on increasing the intake of nutritious and healthy foods like grains, veggies, fruits, beans, etc.
As you are about to discover, the Dash diet can be easy to follow because there are so many dietary options you have at hand.
There are so many healthy, rich and delicious dishes you can consume on a Dash diet and we've gathered the best 250 ones.
But, wait! There's more!

We thought you could use some Dash diet recipes made in one of the most amazing and popular kitchen appliances: the slow cooker.
Slow cookers are simply the future in the kitchen not just because it allows you to work less in the kitchen. Slow cookers are so great because they help you cook healthy dishes using fresh and nutritious ingredients.

So, if you want to reduce the risk of heart disease, cancer, diabetes or even stroke you should consider adopting a healthy diet such as the Dash diet and if you want to cook the best Dash diet dishes you have to use your slow cooker!

Don't trust us! Just check out the recipes collection we've gathered for you!
It's will be a life-changing experience for sure!
Start living a new life with the Dash diet and prepare the best Dash diet recipes in your slow cooker!
Have fun!

Dash Diet Slow Cooker Breakfast Recipes

Delicious Apple Granola Breakfast

Preparation time: 10 minutes
Cooking time: 0 minutes
Servings: 4

Ingredients:
- 2 green apples, peeled, cored and cut into medium chunks
- ½ cup granola
- ½ cup bran flakes
- ¼ cup natural apple juice
- 1 teaspoon stevia
- 2 tablespoons dairy free butter
- ½ teaspoon nutmeg, ground
- 1 teaspoon cinnamon powder

Directions:
In your slow cooker, mix the apples with the granola, bran flakes, apple juice, stevia, butter, nutmeg and cinnamon, toss, cover and cook on Low for 4 hours. Divide into bowls and serve. Enjoy!

Nutrition: calories 200, fat 3, fiber 6, carbs 8, protein 4

Delicious Banana and Coconut Oatmeal

Preparation time: 10 minutes
Cooking time: 7 hours
Servings: 4

Ingredients:
- 2 cups banana, peeled and sliced
- 28 ounces coconut milk
- ½ cup water
- 1 cup old-fashioned rolled oats
- 2 tablespoons stevia
- 1 tablespoon dairy free butter
- ¼ teaspoon nutmeg, ground
- ½ teaspoon cinnamon powder
- ½ teaspoon vanilla extract
- 1 tablespoon flax seed

Directions:
In your slow cooker, combine the banana with the milk, water, oats, stevia, butter, nutmeg, cinnamon, vanilla and flax seed, toss a bit, cover and cook on Low for 7 hours. Divide into bowls and serve.
Enjoy!

Nutrition: calories 231, fat 1, fiber 5, carbs 9, protein 5

Carrot and Zucchini Oatmeal

Preparation time: 10 minutes
Cooking time: 8 hours
Servings: 4

Ingredients:
- ½ cup gluten-free oats
- 1 carrot, grated
- 1 and ½ cups coconut milk
- ¼ zucchini, grated
- ¼ teaspoon nutmeg, ground
- ¼ teaspoon cloves, ground
- ½ teaspoon cinnamon powder
- 2 tablespoons agave nectar
- ¼ cup walnuts, chopped

Directions:
In your slow cooker, combine the oats with the carrot, zucchini, milk, nutmeg, cloves, cinnamon and agave nectar, cover and cook on Low for 8 hours. Divide into bowls, sprinkle walnuts on top and serve.
Enjoy!

Nutrition: calories 211, fat 2, fiber 5, carbs 9, protein 4

Coconut Quinoa Mix

Preparation time: 10 minutes
Cooking time: 4 hours
Servings: 4

Ingredients:
- 3 cups coconut water
- 1 teaspoon vanilla extract
- 1 cup quinoa
- 2 teaspoons honey
- 1/8 coconut flakes
- ¼ cup cranberries
- 1/8 cup almonds, sliced

Directions:
In your slow cooker, mix the coconut water with the quinoa, vanilla, honey, coconut, almonds and cranberries, cover and cook on Low for 4 hours. Stir the quinoa mix, divide it between plates and serve for breakfast.
Enjoy!

Nutrition: calories 217, fat 2, fiber 3, carbs 9, protein 4

Simple Banana Bread

Preparation time: 10 minutes
Cooking time: 4 hours
Servings: 4

Ingredients:
- 2 eggs
- 2 tablespoons olive oil
- 2 cups whole wheat flour
- 1 teaspoon baking powder
- ½ teaspoon baking soda
- 3 bananas, peeled and mashed

Directions:
In a bowl, mix the eggs with the oil, flour, baking powder and baking soda and whisk well. Add bananas, stir the batter, pour it into your greased slow cooker, cover and cook on Low for 4 hours. Slice the bread, divide it between plates and serve.
Enjoy!

Nutrition: calories 251, fat 2, fiber 6, carbs 8, protein 5

Greek Dash Casserole

Preparation time: 10 minutes
Cooking time: 4 hours
Servings: 6

Ingredients:
- 12 eggs, whisked
- Black pepper to the taste
- ½ cup low-fat milk
- 1 tablespoon red onion, chopped
- 1 teaspoon garlic, minced
- 1 cup baby bell mushrooms, sliced
- 2 cups spinach

Directions:
In a bowl, mix the eggs with black pepper, milk, onion, garlic, mushrooms and spinach, toss, pour into your slow cooker, cover and cook on Low for 4 hours. Slice, divide between plates and serve.
Enjoy!

Nutrition: calories 200, fat 3, fiber 7, carbs 9, protein 5

Easy Breakfast Casserole

Preparation time: 10 minutes
Cooking time: 4 hours
Servings: 8

Ingredients:
- 8 eggs
- ¾ cup low-fat milk
- 2 teaspoons mustard
- 1 teaspoon garlic, minced
- 30 ounces hash browns
- ½ yellow onion, chopped
- 2 bell peppers, chopped
- 1 small broccoli head, florets separated
- A pinch of black pepper

Directions:
In a bowl, mix the eggs with the milk, mustard, garlic, hash browns, onion, bell peppers, broccoli and black pepper, stir, pour into your slow cooker, cover and cook on Low for 4 hours. Divide between plates and serve.
Enjoy!

Nutrition: calories 200, fat 4, fiber 7, carbs 8, protein 5

Mexican Dash Diet Eggs

Preparation time: 5 minutes
Cooking time: 2 hours
Servings: 8

Ingredients:
- 10 eggs
- Olive oil cooking spray
- 12 ounces low-fat cheese, shredded
- 1 cup nonfat sour cream
- ½ teaspoon chili powder
- Black pepper to the taste
- 1 garlic clove, minced
- 5 ounces canned green chilies, drained
- 10 ounces tomato sauce, sodium-free

Directions:
In a bowl, mix the eggs with the cheese, sour cream, chili powder, black pepper, garlic, green chilies and tomato sauce, whisk, and pour into your slow cooker after you've greased it with cooking oil, cover and cook on Low for 2 hours. Divide between plates and serve.
Enjoy!

Nutrition: calories 211, fat 2, fiber 5, carbs 8, protein 5

Simple Apple Oatmeal

Preparation time: 5 minutes
Cooking time: 10 hours
Servings: 4

Ingredients:
- 2 teaspoons low-fat butter
- 4 apples, peeled, cored and chopped
- 1 cup coconut sugar
- 1 and ½ tablespoon cinnamon powder
- 2 cups old-fashioned pats
- 4 cups coconut water

Directions:
Grease your slow cooker with the butter, add apples, coconut sugar, cinnamon, oats and water, cover and cook on Low for 10 hours. Stir the oatmeal, divide into bowls and serve.
Enjoy!

Nutrition: calories 211, fat 4, fiber 3, carbs 9, protein 3

Easy Quinoa and Oats

Preparation time: 10 minutes
Cooking time: 7 hours
Servings: 6

Ingredients:
- 1 and ½ cups steel cut oats
- ½ cup quinoa
- 4 cups water
- 2 tablespoons stevia
- 2 tablespoons maple syrup
- ½ teaspoon vanilla extract

Directions:
In your slow cooker, mix the oats with the quinoa, water, stevia, maple syrup and vanilla, cover and cook on Low for 7 hours. Stir the oatmeal, divide it into bowls and serve.
Enjoy!

Nutrition: calories 199, fat 2, fiber 7, carbs 9, protein 3

Easy Pumpkin Oatmeal

Preparation time: 10 minutes
Cooking time: 9 hours
Servings: 4

Ingredients:
- 1 cup steel cut oats
- ½ cup pumpkin puree
- 4 cups water
- Olive oil cooking spray
- ½ cup fat-free milk
- 2 tablespoons stevia
- ½ teaspoon cinnamon powder
- A pinch of cloves, ground
- A pinch of allspice, ground
- A pinch of ginger, ground
- A pinch of nutmeg, ground

Directions:
Grease your slow cooker with the cooking spray, add the oats, the pumpkin puree, water, milk, stevia, cinnamon, cloves, allspice, ginger and nutmeg, cover and cook on Low for 9 hours. Stir the oatmeal, divide it into bowls and serve.
Enjoy!

Nutrition: calories 218, fat 3, fiber 6, carbs 18, protein 7

Raspberry Oatmeal

Preparation time: 10 minutes
Cooking time: 6 hours
Servings: 4

Ingredients:
- 1 tablespoon coconut oil
- 1 cup steel cut oats
- 2 cups water
- 1 cup nonfat milk
- 1 tablespoon stevia
- ½ teaspoon vanilla extract
- 1 cup raspberries
- 4 tablespoons walnuts

Directions:
In your slow cooker, combine the oil with the oats, water, milk, stevia, vanilla, raspberries and walnuts, cover and cook on Low for 6 hours. Divide the oatmeal into bowls and serve.
Enjoy!

Nutrition: calories 187, fat 7, fiber 4, carbs 12, protein 4

Delicious Frittata

Preparation time: 10 minutes
Cooking time: 3 hours
Servings: 6

Ingredients:
- 14 ounces small artichoke hearts, drained
- 12 ounces roasted red peppers, chopped
- 8 eggs, whisked
- ¼ cup green onions, chopped
- A pinch of black pepper
- 4 ounces low-fat cheese, grated

Directions:
In your slow cooker, mix the eggs with the red peppers, artichokes, green onions and black pepper and whisk. Spread the cheese all over, cover and cook on Low for 3 hours. Slice, divide between plates and serve.
Enjoy!

Nutrition: calories 214, fat 3, fiber 7, carbs 12, protein 5

Spinach Frittata

Preparation time: 10 minutes
Cooking time: 2 hours
Servings: 4

Ingredients:
- 1 tablespoon olive oil
- ½ cup yellow onion, chopped
- 1 cup low-fat cheese, shredded
- 3 eggs
- 3 egg whites
- 2 tablespoon low-fat milk
- A pinch of black pepper
- A pinch of white pepper
- 1 cup baby spinach leaves
- 1 tomato, chopped

Directions:
In a bowl, mix the eggs with the egg whites, milk, white and black pepper, spinach and tomato and stir. Grease the slow cooker with the oil, pour eggs mix, spread the cheese on top, cover and cook on Low for 2 hours. Slice the frittata, divide between plates and serve.
Enjoy!

Nutrition: calories 211, fat 2, fiber 6, carbs 15, protein 6

Breakfast Veggie Omelet

Preparation time: 10 minutes
Cooking time: 2 hours
Servings: 4

Ingredients:
- 6 eggs, whisked
- ½ cup low-fat milk
- Black pepper to the taste
- A pinch of chili powder
- A pinch of garlic powder
- 1 cup broccoli florets
- 1 red bell pepper, chopped
- 1 yellow onion, chopped
- Cooking spray
- 1 garlic clove, minced

Directions:
In a bowl, mix the eggs with the milk, black pepper, chili powder, garlic powder, red bell pepper, broccoli, onion and garlic and whisk well. Grease your slow cooker with the cooking spray, spread the eggs mix on the bottom, cover and cook on High for 2 hours. Slice the omelet, divide it between plates and serve.
Enjoy!

Nutrition: calories 182, fat 3, fiber 5, carbs 15, protein 4

Scrambled Eggs

Preparation time: 10 minutes
Cooking time: 8 hours
Servings: 8

Ingredients:
- 12 eggs
- 6 ounces hash browns
- 15 ounces sausage, sliced
- 16 ounces low-fat cheese, shredded
- 1 cup nonfat milk
- 2 drops Tabasco sauce
- Black pepper to the taste

Directions:
In a bowl, mix the eggs with the hash browns, sausage, milk, black pepper and Tabasco and whisk well. Spread this into your slow cooker, spread the cheese on top, cover and cook on Low for 8 hours. Stir the scrambled eggs, divide them between plates and serve.
Enjoy!

Nutrition: calories 211, fat 3, fiber 6, carbs 14, protein 4

Apple and Raisins Oatmeal

Preparation time: 10 minutes
Cooking time: 6 hours
Servings: 4

Ingredients:
- 2 cups almond milk
- 1 tablespoon low-fat butter
- 2 tablespoons stevia
- ½ teaspoon cinnamon powder
- 2 drops vanilla extract
- 1 cup apple, chopped
- ¼ cup raisins
- 1 cup old-fashioned oats
- Cooking spray

Directions:
Grease your slow cooker with the cooking spray, add milk, honey, butter, cinnamon and vanilla and stir. Add oats, apples and raisins, cover and cook on Low for 7 hours. Divide into bowls and serve.
Enjoy!

Nutrition: calories 200, fat 1, fiber 4, carbs 9, protein 4

Delicious Peanut Butter Oats

Preparation time: 10 minutes
Cooking time: 6 hours
Servings: 2

Ingredients:
- 1 cup almond milk
- 2 tablespoon chia seeds
- 4 tablespoons peanut butter
- 1 tablespoon stevia
- 1 cup rolled oats

Directions:
In your slow cooker, mix the oats with the milk, chia, peanut butter and stevia, cover and cook on Low for 6 hours. Stir the oats mix, divide into bowls and serve.
Enjoy!

Nutrition: calories 211, fat 2, fiber 6, carbs 12, protein 5

Orange and Strawberry Breakfast Mix

Preparation time: 5 minutes
Cooking time: 4 hours
Servings: 2

Ingredients:
- 1 cup low-fat milk
- 1 cup orange juice
- 6 ounces low-fat yogurt
- 20 ounces strawberries

Directions:
In your slow cooker, mix orange juice with milk and strawberries, cover and cook on Low for 4 hours. Divide the yogurt into bowls, add the orange and strawberry mix on top and serve.
Enjoy!

Nutrition: calories 180, fat 3, fiber 4, carbs 11, protein 1

Delicious Omelet

Preparation time: 10 minutes
Cooking time: 2 hours
Servings: 4

Ingredients:
- 8 eggs, whisked
- Cooking spray
- Salt and black pepper to the taste
- 2 tablespoons chives, chopped
- A pinch of cayenne pepper
- 2 ounces low-fat cheddar cheese, grated
- 2 cups spinach, torn

For the red pepper relish:
- 2 tablespoons green onion, chopped
- 1 cup red pepper, chopped
- 1 tablespoon vinegar

Directions:
In a bowl, mix eggs with salt, pepper, cayenne and chives and stir well. Grease your slow cooker with cooking spray, add eggs mix and spread. Add spinach and cheese, toss, cover and cook on High for 2 hours. In a bowl, mix red pepper with green onions, black pepper to the taste and the vinegar and stir well. Slice the omelet, divide it between plates, top with the relish and serve for breakfast.
Enjoy!

Nutrition: calories 200, fat 4, fiber 5, carbs 13, protein 5

Fruits and Cereals Mix

Preparation time: 10 minutes
Cooking time: 6 hours
Servings: 6

Ingredients:
- 4 cups mixed orange, apple, grapes and pineapple pieces
- 2 tablespoons honey
- ½ cup whole wheat and barley cereals
- 12 ounces almond milk
- ¼ cup coconut, toasted and shredded

Directions:
In your slow cooker, mix the fruits with the honey, cereals and milk, cover and cook on Low for 6 hours. Divide into bowls, sprinkle coconut on top and serve.
Enjoy!

Nutrition: calories 190, fat 3, fiber 3, carbs 6, protein 3

Breakfast Berries Compote

Preparation time: 10 minutes
Cooking time: 4 hours
Servings: 4

Ingredients:
- 2 tablespoons white wine vinegar
- 2 cups blueberries
- ½ cup palm sugar
- 2 tablespoons lemon juice
- ½ teaspoon lemon zest, grated
- 2 peaches, pitted, peeled and cut into wedges
- 1 and ½ cups raspberries
- 1 and ½ cups blackberries

Directions:
In your slow cooker, mix blueberries with sugar, vinegar, lemon juice and lemon zest, cover and cook on Low for 4 hours. Divide this into 4 bowl, top with raspberries, blackberries and peach wedges and serve for breakfast.
Enjoy!

Nutrition: calories 170, fat 1, fiber 1, carbs 8, protein 4

Apples and Dates Oatmeal

Preparation time: 10 minutes
Cooking time: 7 hours
Servings: 4

Ingredients:
- 4 cups water
- 3 cups rolled oats
- 3 cups whole grain cereal flakes
- 1 cup apples, dried and chopped
- 1 cup dates, dried and chopped
- 1 cup walnuts, chopped
- 2 tablespoons cinnamon powder
- 1 cup coconut sugar
- 1 teaspoon cloves, ground
- 1 tablespoon ginger, ground
- 1 teaspoon turmeric powder

Directions:
In your slow cooker, mix the water with the oats, cereal flakes, apples, dates, walnuts, cinnamon, sugar, cloves, ginger and turmeric, cover and cook on Low for 7 hours. Divide into bowls and serve.
Enjoy!

Nutrition: calories 150, fat 3, fiber 6, carbs 10, protein 3

Scrambled Eggs and Veggies

Preparation time: 10 minutes
Cooking time: 8 hours
Servings: 4

Ingredients:
- 3 eggs
- ¼ cup green bell pepper, chopped
- ¾ cup tomato, chopped
- Cooking spray
- ¼ cup green onions, chopped
- ¼ cup fat-free milk
- A pinch of black pepper
- A splash of hot pepper

Directions:
In a bowl, mix the eggs with the bell pepper, tomato, onions, milk, black pepper and hot pepper and stir. Grease the slow cooker with the cooking spray, add eggs mix, cover and cook on Low for 8 hours. Stir the eggs, divide them between plates and serve.
Enjoy!

Nutrition: calories 190, fat 2, fiber 3, carbs 12, protein 5

Mexican Casserole

Preparation time: 10 minutes
Cooking time: 4 hours
Servings: 8

Ingredients:
- ¾ cup canned enchilada sauce
- 15 ounces canned black beans, drained and rinsed
- 8 ounces canned green chili peppers, chopped
- A splash of hot pepper sauce
- ½ cup green onions, chopped
- Cooking spray
- 1 cup low-fat cheddar cheese, grated
- 2 garlic cloves, minced
- 3 egg whites
- 2 tablespoons whole wheat flour
- 3 egg yolks
- ½ cup fat-free milk
- 1 tablespoon cilantro, chopped

Directions:
Grease your slow cooker with cooking spray and add beans, chili peppers, enchilada sauce, green onions, pepper sauce, salt, garlic and cheese. In a bowl, beat egg whites with a mixer. In a separate bowl, mix egg yolks with salt and flour and whisk well. Add egg whites, milk and cilantro and whisk well again. Pour this over beans mix, spread well, cover and cook on Low for 4 hours. Slice, divide between plates and serve for breakfast.
Enjoy!

Nutrition: calories 240, fat 4, fiber 3, carbs 6, protein 6

Shrimp Frittata

Preparation time: 10 minutes
Cooking time: 4 hours
Servings: 4

Ingredients:
- 4 ounces shrimp, peeled, deveined and cut into halves horizontally
- 2 eggs
- 4 ounces canned artichokes, drained and chopped
- ¼ cup fat-free milk
- A pinch of black pepper
- A pinch of garlic powder
- ¼ cup green onions, chopped
- Cooking spray
- 3 tablespoons low-fat cheddar cheese, grated
- 8 cherry tomatoes, halved
- 1 tablespoon parsley, chopped

Directions:
In a bowl, mix the eggs with milk, black pepper, garlic powder and green onions and stir well. Grease your slow cooker with the cooking spray, add eggs mix, cover and cook on Low for 3 hours and 30 minutes. Add shrimp, artichokes, cheddar cheese, tomatoes and parsley on top, cover and cook on Low for 30 minutes. Divide frittata between plates and serve for breakfast.
Enjoy!

Nutrition: calories 200, fat 2, fiber 3, carbs 13, protein 4

Tofu Scramble

Preparation time: 10 minutes
Cooking time: 5 hours
Servings: 4

Ingredients:
- 18 ounces package firm tofu, drained well, pat dried and crumbled
- 2 poblano chili peppers, chopped
- 1 tablespoon olive oil
- 2 garlic cloves, minced
- ½ cup onion, chopped
- 1 teaspoon chili powder
- ½ teaspoon oregano, dried
- ½ teaspoon cumin, ground
- 2 tomatoes, peeled and chopped
- 1 tablespoon lime juice
- 1 tablespoon cilantro, chopped

Directions:
Grease the slow cooker with the oil and add chili peppers, garlic and onion. Also add chili powder, oregano and cumin and stir. Add tofu, tomatoes, lime juice and cilantro, stir well again, cover and cook on Low for 5 hours. Divide the scramble between plates and serve.
Enjoy!

Nutrition: calories 200, fat 3, fiber 2, carbs 14, protein 5

Squash and Apples Breakfast Mix

Preparation time: 10 minutes
Cooking time: 6 hours
Servings: 2

Ingredients:
- 1 big apple, cored, peeled and cut into wedges
- 1 acorn squash, halved, deseeded and cubed
- 2 tablespoons stevia
- 2 teaspoons avocado oil

Directions:
Grease your slow cooker with the oil, add apple, squash and stevia, toss, cover and cook on Low for 6 hours. Divide into bowls and serve for breakfast.
Enjoy!

Nutrition: calories 200, fat 5, fiber 6, carbs 13, protein 5

Corn Pudding

Preparation time: 10 minutes
Cooking time: 6 hours
Servings: 8

Ingredients:
- 3 cups fat-free milk
- 3 cups water
- ¼ cup maple syrup
- 2 cups cornmeal
- A pinch of nutmeg, ground
- ¼ teaspoon cinnamon powder
- A pinch of cloves, ground
- ½ cup raisins
- A pinch of ginger, grated

Directions:
In your slow cooker, mix the water with the milk and cornmeal and stir. Add raisins, maple syrup, nutmeg, cinnamon, cloves and ginger, stir, cover, cook on Low for 6 hours. Divide between plates and serve.
Enjoy!

Nutrition: calories 170, fat 1, fiber 2, carbs 14, protein 7

Sweet Potatoes Mix

Preparation time: 10 minutes
Cooking time: 7 hours
Servings: 8

Ingredients:
- 2 tablespoons stevia
- ¼ cup water
- 1 tablespoon olive oil
- 2 tablespoons honey
- 4 sweet potatoes, peeled and cut into wedges
- Black pepper to the taste
- A pinch of rosemary, dried

Directions:
In your slow cooker, mix the potatoes with the oil, black pepper, rosemary, water, honey and stevia, toss, cover and cook on Low for 7 hours. Divide between plates and serve for breakfast.
Enjoy!

Nutrition: calories 200, fat 3, fiber 4, carbs 12, protein 2

Almond and Cherries Oats

Preparation time: 10 minutes
Cooking time: 8 hours
Servings: 4

Ingredients:
- 2 cups almond milk
- 1 cup steel cut oats
- 2 cups water
- 1/3 cup cherries, dried
- 2 tablespoons cocoa powder
- ¼ cup stevia
- ½ teaspoon almond extract

Directions:
In your slow cooker, mix almond milk with oats, water, dried cherries, cocoa powder, stevia and the almond extract, stir, cover and cook on Low for 8 hours. Divide the oats into bowls and serve for breakfast.
Enjoy!

Nutrition: calories 202, fat 7, fiber 7, carbs 12, protein 6

Cranberry Toast

Preparation time: 10 minutes
Cooking time: 5 hours
Servings: 4

Ingredients:
- 1 tablespoon chia seeds
- ½ tablespoon agave nectar
- 1 cup almond milk
- ½ teaspoon vanilla extract
- ½ teaspoon cinnamon powder
- 4 whole wheat bread slices, cubed
- 1 tablespoon coconut oil

Directions:
Add coconut oil to your slow cooker, also add bread cubes and toss them. Also add milk, chia, vanilla, agave nectar and cinnamon, toss, cover, cook on Low for 5 hours, divide into bowls and serve for breakfast.
Enjoy!

Nutrition: calories 201, fat 4, fiber 7, carbs 14, protein 4

Easy Burrito Bowls

Preparation time: 10 minutes
Cooking time: 6 hours
Servings: 8

Ingredients:

- 16 ounces tofu, crumbled
- 1 green bell pepper, chopped
- ¼ cup scallions, chopped
- 15 ounces canned black beans, drained and rinsed
- 1 cup tomato sauce, sodium free
- ½ cup water
- ¼ teaspoon cumin, ground
- ½ teaspoon turmeric powder
- ½ teaspoon sweet paprika
- A pinch of black pepper
- ¼ teaspoon chili powder
- 3 cups spinach leaves, torn

Directions:
In your slow cooker, mix tofu with bell pepper, scallions, black beans, salsa, water, cumin, turmeric, paprika, salt, pepper and chili powder, stir, cover and cook on Low for 6 hours. Add spinach, toss well, divide into bowls and serve for breakfast.
Enjoy!

Nutrition: calories 211, fat 4, fiber 7, carbs 14, protein 4

Spiced Coconut Oats

Preparation time: 10 minutes
Cooking time: 4 hours
Servings: 6

Ingredients:

- 1 and ½ cups water
- 1 and ½ cups coconut milk
- 2 apples, cored, peeled and chopped
- 1 cup steel cut oats
- ½ teaspoon cinnamon powder
- ¼ teaspoon nutmeg, ground
- ¼ teaspoon allspice, ground
- ¼ teaspoon ginger powder
- ¼ teaspoon cardamom, ground
- 1 tablespoon flax seed, ground
- 2 teaspoons vanilla extract
- 2 teaspoons stevia
- Cooking spray

Directions:
Spray your slow cooker with cooking spray, add apple pieces, milk, water, cinnamon, oats, allspice, nutmeg, and cardamom, ginger, vanilla, flax seeds and stevia, cover and cook on Low for 4 hours. Stir the oatmeal, divide into bowls and serve for breakfast.
Enjoy!

Nutrition: calories 172, fat 3, fiber 7, carbs 12, protein 5

Easy Carrot Oatmeal

Preparation time: 10 minutes
Cooking time: 7 hours
Servings: 4

Ingredients:
- 2 cups coconut milk
- ½ cup steel cut oats
- 1 cup carrots, shredded
- 1 teaspoon cardamom, ground
- ½ teaspoon agave nectar
- A pinch of saffron powder
- Cooking spray

Directions:
Spray your slow cooker with cooking spray; add milk, oats, carrots, cardamom and agave nectar, stir, cover and cook on Low for 7 hours. Stir oatmeal, divide into bowls, sprinkle saffron on top and serve for breakfast.
Enjoy!

Nutrition: calories 182, fat 7, fiber 4, carbs 8, protein 3

Simple Blueberries Oatmeal

Preparation time: 10 minutes
Cooking time: 8 hours
Servings: 4

Ingredients:
- 1 cup blueberries
- 1 cup steel cut oats
- 1 cup coconut milk
- 2 tablespoons agave nectar
- ½ teaspoon vanilla extract
- Coconut flakes for serving
- Cooking spray

Directions:
Spray your slow cooker with cooking spray, add oats, milk, agave nectar, vanilla and blueberries, toss, cover and cook on Low for 8 hours. Divide the oatmeal into bowls, sprinkle coconut flakes on top and serve.
Enjoy!

Nutrition: calories 202, fat 6, fiber 8, carbs 12, protein 6

Tofu and Veggies Frittata

Preparation time: 10 minutes
Cooking time: 6 hours
Servings: 4

Ingredients:
- 1 pound firm tofu, drained, pressed and crumbled
- 2 tablespoons olive oil
- 1 yellow onion, chopped
- ¼ teaspoon turmeric powder
- 3 tablespoons garlic, minced
- 1 red bell pepper, chopped
- ½ cup kalamata olives, pitted and halved
- 1 teaspoon basil, dried
- 1 teaspoon oregano, dried
- 1 tablespoon lemon juice
- Black pepper to the taste

Directions:
Add the oil to your slow cooker and spread the crumbled tofu. Add onion, turmeric, garlic, bell pepper, olives, basil, oregano, lemon juice and pepper, toss a bit, cover and cook on Low for 6 hours. Divide frittata between plates and serve for breakfast.
Enjoy!

Nutrition: calories 201, fat 4, fiber 7, carbs 10, protein 6

Chia Pudding

Preparation time: 10 minutes
Cooking time: 2 hours
Servings: 4

Ingredients:
- ½ cup coconut chia granola
- ½ cup chia seeds
- 2 cups coconut milk
- 2 tablespoons coconut, shredded and unsweetened
- ¼ cup maple syrup
- ½ teaspoon cinnamon powder
- 2 teaspoons cocoa powder
- ½ teaspoon vanilla extract

Directions:
In your slow cooker, mix chia granola with chia seeds, coconut milk, coconut, maple syrup, cinnamon, cocoa powder and vanilla, toss, cover and cook on High for 2 hours. Divide chia pudding into bowls and serve for breakfast.
Enjoy!

Nutrition: calories 201, fat 4, fiber 8, carbs 11, protein 4

Breakfast Potatoes

Preparation time: 10 minutes
Cooking time: 4 hours
Servings: 8

Ingredients:
- Cooking spray
- 2 pounds gold potatoes, halved and sliced
- 1 yellow onion, cut into medium wedges
- 12 ounces coconut milk
- 1 cup tofu, crumbled
- Black pepper to the taste
- 1 tablespoons parsley, chopped

Directions:
Coat your slow cooker with cooking spray and arrange half of the potatoes on the bottom. Layer half of the onion wedges and half of the coconut milk, tofu and pepper. Add the rest of the potatoes, onion wedges, coconut milk, tofu and stock, cover and cook on High for 4 hours. Sprinkle parsley on top, divide the whole mix between plates and serve.
Enjoy!

Nutrition: calories 200, fat 14, fiber 4, carbs 13, protein 12

Breakfast Nuts and Squash Bowls

Preparation time: 10 minutes
Cooking time: 8 hours
Servings: 4

Ingredients:
- ½ cup almonds
- ½ cup walnuts
- A splash of water
- 2 apples, peeled, cored and cubed
- 1 butternut squash, peeled and cubed
- 1 teaspoon cinnamon powder
- 1 tablespoon stevia
- ½ teaspoon nutmeg, ground
- 1 cup coconut milk

Directions:
Put almonds and walnuts in your blender, add a splash of water, blend really well and transfer to your slow cooker. Add apples, squash, cinnamon, stevia, nutmeg and coconut milk, stir, cover and cook on Low for 8 hours. Stir, divide into bowls and serve.
Enjoy!

Nutrition: calories 170, fat 1, fiber 2, carbs 8, protein 5

Leeks, Kale and Sweet Potato Mix

Preparation time: 10 minutes
Cooking time: 6 hours and 10 minutes
Servings: 4

Ingredients:
- 1 and 1/3 cups leek, chopped
- 2 tablespoons olive oil
- 1 cup kale, chopped
- 2 teaspoons garlic, minced
- 8 eggs
- 2/3 cup sweet potato, grated
- 1 and ½ cups sausage, chopped

Directions:
Heat up a pan with the oil over medium- high heat; add sausage, stir, and brown for 2-3 minutes and transfer to your slow cooker. Add garlic, sweet potatoes, kale and crack the eggs. Stir, cover, cook on Low for 6 hours, divide between plates and serve.
Enjoy!

Nutrition: calories 210, fat 2, fiber 2, carbs 13, protein 10

Egg Casserole

Preparation time: 10 minutes
Cooking time: 8 hours and 10 minutes
Servings: 4

Ingredients:
- 1 red onion, chopped
- 3 sausage links, sliced
- 1 red bell pepper, chopped
- 2 sweet potatoes, grated
- 12 eggs
- 2 garlic cloves, minced
- 1 tablespoon olive oil
- 1 teaspoon dill, chopped
- 1 cup coconut milk
- A pinch of red pepper, crushed
- Black pepper to the taste

Directions:
Heat up a pan with the oil over medium- high heat, add garlic, bell pepper and onion, stir and cook for 5 minutes. Add grated sweet potato, red pepper and black pepper, stir and cook for 2 minutes more. Transfer half of this to your slow cooker and spread on the bottom. In a bowl, mix eggs with coconut milk and whisk well. Pour half of the eggs over the veggies, add sausage, add another veggie layer and top with the rest of the eggs. Sprinkle dill all over, cover, cook on Low for 8 hours, slice and serve for breakfast.
Enjoy!

Nutrition: calories 240, fat 2, fiber 3, carbs 10, protein 8

Maple Apples

Preparation time: 10 minutes
Cooking time: 1 hour and 30 minutes
Servings: 4

Ingredients:
- ½ cup maple syrup
- ¼ cup figs
- 1 teaspoon stevia
- ¼ cup walnuts, chopped
- 1 teaspoon lemon zest, grated
- ½ teaspoon orange zest, grated
- 1 teaspoon cinnamon powder
- ¼ teaspoon nutmeg, ground
- 1 tablespoon lemon juice
- 1 tablespoon avocado oil
- ½ cup water
- 4 apples, cored and tops cut off

Directions:
In a bowl, mix maple syrup with figs, stevia, walnuts, lemon and orange zest, half of the cinnamon, nutmeg, lemon juice and the oil, whisk really well and stuff apples with this mix. Add the water to your slow cooker, add the rest of the cinnamon, stir, add apples inside, cover and cook on High for 1 hour and 30 minutes. Divide apples between plates and serve for breakfast. Enjoy!

Nutrition: calories 199, fat 4, fiber 7, carbs 12, protein 4

Apples and Sauce

Preparation time: 10 minutes
Cooking time: 4 hours
Servings: 4

Ingredients:
- 1/3 cup avocado oil
- 1 tablespoon lemon juice
- ¼ cup cane juice
- ½ teaspoon cinnamon powder
- 1 teaspoon vanilla extract
- 5 apples, cored, peeled and cubed

Directions:
In your slow cooker, mix coconut oil with cane juice, lemon juice, cinnamon and vanilla and whisk well. Add apple cubes, toss well, cover, cook on High for 4 hours, divide into bowls and serve for breakfast.
Enjoy!

Nutrition: calories 200, fat 4, fiber 6, carbs 12, protein 4

Sweet Potato and Sausage Pie

Preparation time: 10 minutes
Cooking time: 8 hours
Servings: 4

Ingredients:
- 1 sweet potato, shredded
- 8 eggs, whisked
- 2 teaspoons coconut oil, melted
- 1 pound sausage, crumbled
- 1 tablespoon garlic powder
- 1 yellow onion, chopped
- 2 teaspoons basil, dried
- 2 red bell peppers, chopped
- Black pepper to the taste

Directions:
Grease your slow cooker with the oil, add sweet potatoes, sausage, garlic powder, bell pepper, onion, basil, salt and pepper. Add the eggs, toss, cover, cook on Low for 8 hours, divide between plates and serve.
Enjoy!

Nutrition: calories 224, fat 7, fiber 8, carbs 14, protein 6

Pumpkin Butter

Preparation time: 10 minutes
Cooking time: 4 hours
Servings: 8

Ingredients:
- 30 ounces pumpkin puree
- ½ cup apple cider
- 1 cup coconut sugar
- 1 teaspoon vanilla extract
- 1 teaspoon cinnamon powder
- 1 teaspoon nutmeg, ground
- 2 teaspoon lemon juice
- 1 teaspoon ginger, grated
- ¼ teaspoon cloves, ground
- ¼ teaspoon allspice, ground

Directions:
In your slow cooker, mix pumpkin puree with apple cider, coconut sugar, vanilla extract, cinnamon, nutmeg, lemon juice, ginger, cloves and allspice, stir, cover and cook on Low for 4 hours. Blend using an immersion blender and serve for breakfast.
Enjoy!

Nutrition: calories 202, fat 3, fiber 3, carbs 9, protein 3

Pineapple and Carrot Mix

Preparation time: 10 minutes
Cooking time: 6 hours
Servings: 10

Ingredients:
- 1 cup raisins
- 6 cups water
- 23 ounces natural applesauce
- 2 tablespoons stevia
- 2 tablespoons cinnamon powder
- 14 ounces carrots, shredded
- 8 ounces canned pineapple, crushed
- 1 tablespoon pumpkin pie spice

Directions:
In your slow cooker, mix carrots with applesauce, raisins, stevia, cinnamon, pineapple and pumpkin pie spice, stir, cover, cook on Low for 6 hours, divide into bowls and serve for breakfast.
Enjoy!

Nutrition: calories 179, fat 2, fiber 3, carbs 15, protein 4

Spinach Pie

Preparation time: 10 minutes
Cooking time: 4 hours
Servings: 4

Ingredients:
- 10 ounces spinach
- 2 cups baby Bella mushrooms, chopped
- 1 red bell pepper, chopped
- 1 and ½ cups low-fat cheese, shredded
- 8 eggs
- 1 cup coconut cream
- 2 tablespoons chives, chopped
- A pinch of black pepper
- ½ cup almond flour
- ¼ teaspoons baking soda
- Cooking spray

Directions:
In a bowl, combine the eggs with coconut cream, chives and pepper and whisk. Add almond flour, baking soda, cheese, bell pepper, mushrooms and spinach, toss, transfer to your slow cooker greased with cooking spray, cover and cook on Low for 4 hours. Slice, divide between plates and serve for breakfast.
Enjoy!

Nutrition: calories 201, fat 6, fiber 6, carbs 8, protein 5

Creamy Veggie Omelet

Preparation time: 10 minutes
Cooking time: 3 hours
Servings: 4

Ingredients:
- Cooking spray
- 6 eggs
- 1 tablespoon coconut milk
- ½ red bell pepper, chopped
- ½ green bell pepper, chopped
- 1 small yellow onion, chopped
- 1 cup low-fat cheese, shredded
- A pinch of salt and black pepper

Directions:
Grease your slow cooker with cooking spray and spread onion, red and green bell pepper on the bottom. In a bowl, mix the eggs with pepper, cheese and milk, whisk well, pour into the slow cooker, cover, cook on High for 3 hours, divide between plates and serve for breakfast.
Enjoy!

Nutrition: calories 202, fat 6, fiber 5, carbs 8, protein 6

Salmon Omelet

Preparation time: 10 minutes
Cooking time: 3 hours and 40 minutes
Servings: 3

Ingredients:
- 4 eggs, whisked
- ½ teaspoon olive oil
- A pinch black pepper
- 4 ounces smoked salmon, chopped
- 1 cup almond milk
- ½ cup cashews, soaked, drained
- ¼ cup green onions, chopped
- 1 teaspoon garlic powder
- 1 tablespoon lemon juice

Directions:
In your blender, mix cashews with milk, garlic powder, lemon juice, green onions and pepper, blend really well and leave aside. Drizzle the oil in your slow cooker, add eggs, whisk, cover and cook on Low for 3 hours. Add salmon, toss, cover, cook on Low for 40 minutes more, divide between plates, drizzle green onions sauce all over and serve.
Enjoy!

Nutrition: calories 190, fat 10, fiber 2, carbs 6, protein 5

Chicken Omelet

Preparation time: 10 minutes
Cooking time: 3 hours
Servings: 2

Ingredients:
- 1-ounce rotisserie chicken, shredded
- 1 teaspoon mustard
- 1 tablespoon avocado mayonnaise
- 1 tomato, chopped
- 4 eggs, whisked
- 1 small avocado, pitted, peeled and chopped
- Black pepper to the taste

Directions:
In a bowl, mix the eggs with chicken, avocado, tomato, mayo and mustard, toss, transfer to your slow cooker, cover, cook on Low for 3 hours, divide between plates and serve.
Enjoy!

Nutrition: calories 220, fat 9, fiber 6, carbs 4, protein 6

Dash Diet Slow Cooker Main Dish Recipes

Chicken Tacos

Preparation time: 10 minutes
Cooking time: 6 hours and 30 minutes
Servings: 6

Ingredients:
- 1 and ½ pounds chicken breast halves, boneless and skinless
- 1 teaspoon lemon zest, grated
- 3 tablespoons lime juice
- 1 tablespoon chili powder
- 1 cup corn
- 1 cup salsa
- 12 fat-free tortillas
- Low-fat sour cream for serving
- Shredded lettuce for serving

Directions:
In a bowl, mix the limejuice with chili powder and lemon zest and whisk. Put the chicken in your slow cooker, add lime mix, toss, cover and cook on Low for 6 hours. Transfer chicken to a cutting board, shred using 2 forks and return to the pot. Add salsa and corn, cover and cook on Low for 30 minutes more. Divide this mix on each tortilla, also add sour cream and lettuce wrap and serve.
Enjoy!

Nutrition: calories 238, fat 3, fiber 3, carbs 28, protein 15

Quinoa Casserole

Preparation time: 10 minutes
Cooking time: 4 hours
Servings: 4

Ingredients:
- 12 ounces tomatillos, chopped
- 1 red bell pepper, chopped
- 1 pint cherry tomatoes, chopped
- ½ cup white onion, chopped
- 1 cup quinoa
- 1 tablespoon lime juice
-
- 1 cup low-fat Swiss cheese, shredded
- 2 pounds yellow summer squash, cubed
- 2 tablespoon oregano, chopped
- A pinch of black pepper
- Cooking spray

Directions:
In a bowl, mix the tomatoes with tomatillos, onion, limejuice and black pepper and toss. Grease your slow cooker with the cooking spray and add quinoa. Add half of the cheese and the squash and spread. Add the rest of the cheese and the tomatillo mix, spread, cover and cook on Low for 4 hours. Divide between plates, sprinkle oregano on top and serve.
Enjoy!

Nutrition: calories 211, fat 3, fiber 6, carbs 15, protein 4

Quinoa Curry

Preparation time: 10 minutes
Cooking time: 4 hours
Servings: 6

Ingredients:
- 1 sweet potato, chopped
- 2 cups green beans, halved
- 1 carrot, chopped
- 1 small yellow onion, chopped
- 15 ounces canned chickpeas, drained and rinsed
- 28 ounces canned tomatoes, chopped
- 28 ounces coconut milk
- ¼ cup quinoa
- 2 garlic cloves, minced
- 1 tablespoon ginger, grated
- 1 teaspoon turmeric powder
- 2 teaspoons tamari sauce
- 1 and ½ cups water
- 1 teaspoon chili flakes

Directions:
In your slow cooker, combine the potato with green beans, carrot, onion, chickpeas, tomatoes, coconut milk, quinoa, garlic, ginger, turmeric, tamari, water and chili flakes, toss, cover and cook on Low for 4 hours. Divide into bowls and serve.
Enjoy!

Nutrition: calories 211, fat 4, fiber 6, carbs 14, protein 4

Delicious Black Bean Chili

Preparation time: 10 minutes
Cooking time: 4 hours
Servings: 4

Ingredients:
- 1 and ½ cups red bell pepper, chopped
- 1 cup yellow onion, chopped
- 1 and ½ cups mushrooms, sliced
- 1 tablespoon olive oil
- 1 tablespoon chili powder
- 2 garlic cloves, minced
- 1 teaspoon chipotle chili pepper, chopped
- ½ teaspoon cumin, ground
- 16 ounces canned black beans, drained and rinsed
- 2 tablespoons cilantro, chopped
- 1 cup tomatoes, chopped

Directions:
In your slow cooker, combine the red bell peppers with onion, mushrooms, oil, chili powder, garlic, chili pepper, cumin, black beans and tomatoes, stir, cover and cook on High for 4 hours. Divide into bowls, sprinkle cilantro on top and serve.
Enjoy!

Nutrition: calories 211, fat 3, fiber 5, carbs 22, protein 5

Chicken and Veggies

Preparation time: 10 minutes
Cooking time: 4 hours
Servings: 4

Ingredients:
- 2 pounds chicken breasts, skinless and boneless
- 4 cups red potatoes, cubed
- ½ pounds green beans, trimmed
- ¼ cup olive oil
- 1/3 cup lemon juice
- 1 teaspoon oregano, dried
- 1 teaspoon cilantro, dried
- A pinch of black pepper
- 2 garlic cloves, minced
- ¼ teaspoon onion powder

Directions:
Put the chicken breasts in your slow cooker and add green beans and potatoes on top. In a bowl, mix lemon juice with oil, cilantro, black pepper, oregano, and garlic and onion powder and whisk well. Pour this into the slow cooker, cover and cook on High for 4 hours. Divide chicken and veggies between plates and serve.
Enjoy!

Nutrition: calories 211, fat 3, fiber 6, carbs 16, protein 5

Succulent Pork Roast

Preparation time: 10 minutes
Cooking time: 8 hours
Servings: 8

Ingredients:
- 2 pounds pork shoulder roast, boneless
- 1/3 cup low sodium veggie stock
- ½ teaspoon garlic powder
- 1 tablespoon sage, dried
- ¼ cup balsamic vinegar
- 1 tablespoon low sodium Worcestershire sauce
- 1 tablespoon honey

Directions:
Put the roast in your slow cooker and pour the stock over it. In a bowl, mix sage with garlic powder, vinegar, Worcestershire sauce and honey, whisk well, pour into the slow cooker as well, cover and cook on Low for 8 hours. Shred the meat, divide it between plates, drizzle cooking juices all over and serve.
Enjoy!

Nutrition: calories 214, fat 12, fiber 1, carbs 5, protein 21

Turkey Chili

Preparation time: 10 minutes
Cooking time: 8 hours
Servings: 6

Ingredients:
- 2 tablespoons chili powder
- 1 tablespoon garlic powder
- 3 tablespoons onion powder
- ¼ cup cumin, ground
- 2 tablespoons oregano, chopped
- 2 tablespoons sweet paprika
- 1 tablespoon sriracha sauce
- 1 pound turkey meat, ground
- 1 garlic clove, minced
- 1 yellow onion, chopped
- 1 and ½ cup corn
- 1 red bell pepper, chopped
- 1 green bell pepper, chopped
- 28 ounces canned tomatoes, no-salt-added, crushed
- 15 ounces canned kidney beans, no-salt-added, drained and rinsed
- 15 ounces canned black beans, no-salt-added, drained and rinsed
- 9 ounces tomato sauce, no-salt-added

Directions:
In a bowl, mix chili powder with garlic powder, onion powder, cumin, oregano, paprika and sriracha sauce and whisk well. Put the meat in your slow cooker, add spice mix and toss well. Also, add garlic, onion, corn, red and green bell pepper, tomatoes, kidney beans, black beans and tomato sauce, toss, cover and cook on Low for 8 hours. Divide into bowls and serve.
Enjoy!

Nutrition: calories 211, fat 2, fiber 5, carbs 12, protein 17

Easy Pulled Chicken

Preparation time: 10 minutes
Cooking time: 5 hours
Servings: 4

Ingredients:
- 8 ounces tomato sauce, no-salt-added
- 4 ounces canned green chilies, drained and chopped
- 2 tablespoons honey
- 3 tablespoons cider vinegar
- 1 tablespoon sweet paprika
- 1 tablespoon tomato paste
- 1 tablespoon Worcestershire sauce
- 2 teaspoons dried mustard
- 1 teaspoon chipotle chili, dried and ground
- 2 and ½ pounds chicken thighs, boneless and skinless
- 1 yellow onion, chopped
- 1 garlic clove, minced

Directions:
In a bowl, mix the tomato sauce with green chilies, honey, vinegar, paprika, tomato paste, Worcestershire sauce, dried mustard and chipotle chili and whisk really well. Pour this into your slow cooker, add chicken thighs, onion and garlic, toss, cover and cook on Low for 5 hours. Shred the meat using 2 forks, divide everything between plates and serve.
Enjoy!

Nutrition: calories 211, fat 3, fiber 7, carbs 14, protein 8

Mediterranean Chicken

Preparation time: 10 minutes
Cooking time: 2 hours and 30 minutes
Servings: 4

Ingredients:

- 1 pound chicken breasts, skinless and boneless
- 2 tomatoes, chopped
- 1 cup low-sodium chicken stock
- ½ red bell pepper, chopped
- 1 yellow onion, sliced
- Zest of 1 lemon, grated
- Juice of 1 lemon
- Black pepper to the taste
- ¾ cup whole wheat orzo
- ½ cup black olives, pitted
- 2 tablespoons scallions, chopped

Directions:
In your slow cooker, mix chicken with tomatoes, stock, bell pepper, onion, lemon zest, lemon juice and black pepper to the taste, cover and cook on High for 2 hours. Add black olives and orzo, toss, cover, cook on high for 30 minutes more, divide everything between plates and serve with chopped scallions on top.
Enjoy!

Nutrition: calories 211, fat 3, fiber 4, carbs 12, protein 4

Delicious Veggie Soup

Preparation time: 10 minutes
Cooking time: 9 hours and 30 minutes
Servings: 6

Ingredients:

- 15 ounces canned kidney beans, no-salt-added, drained and rinsed
- ½ cup pearl barley
- ½ cup corn
- 14 ounces canned tomatoes, no-salt-added and drained
- 1 cup mushrooms, sliced
- 1 carrot, sliced
- 1 cup yellow onion, chopped
- 1 celery stalk, chopped
- 3 garlic cloves, minced
- ½ cup peas
- ½ cup green beans
- 2 teaspoons oregano, dried
- Black pepper to the taste
- 14 ounces low-sodium chicken stock
- 3 cups fat-free milk
- ¼ cup parsley, chopped

Directions:
In your slow cooker, mix the kidney beans with barley, corn, tomatoes, mushrooms, carrot, onion, celery, garlic, peas, green beans, oregano, black pepper and stock, stir, cover and cook on Low for 9 hours. Add milk and parsley, stir, cover, cook on Low for 30 minutes more, ladle into bowls and serve.
Enjoy!

Nutrition: calories 231, fat 2, fiber 7, carbs 14, protein 5

Chicken and Rice Soup

Preparation time: 10 minutes
Cooking time: 8 hours and 30 minutes
Servings: 4

Ingredients:
- 2 yellow onions, chopped
- 4 garlic clove, minced
- 1 tablespoon olive oil
- 1 tablespoon salt-free tomato paste
- ½ teaspoon thyme, dried
- 8 cups low-sodium chicken stock
- 3 carrots, chopped
- 8 ounces corn
- 2 celery ribs, sliced
- 2 bay leaves
- 2 pounds chicken thighs, skinless and boneless
- 1 cup wild rice
- 2 tablespoons cornstarch
- 2 tablespoon parsley, chopped
- 2 tablespoons water
- 1 tablespoon sriracha

Directions:
In your slow cooker, mix the onions with garlic, oil, tomato paste, thyme, stock, carrots, corn, celery, bay leaves and chicken thighs, cover and cook on Low for 8 hours. Add cornstarch mixed with water, sriracha and rice, stir, cover and cook on Low for 30 minutes more. Ladle soup into bowls, discard bay leaves, sprinkle parsley on top and serve.
Enjoy!

Nutrition: calories 211, fat 3, fiber 7, carbs 17, protein 4

Delicious Black Bean Soup

Preparation time: 10 minutes
Cooking time: 8 hours and 5 minutes
Servings: 4

Ingredients:
- 1 tablespoon olive oil
- 1 yellow onion, chopped
- 4 garlic cloves, minced
- 1 yellow bell pepper, chopped
- 1 red bell pepper, chopped
- 50 ounces canned black beans, no-salt-added, drained and rinsed
- 1 teaspoon cumin, ground
- 4 cups water
- A pinch of black pepper
- 4 cups low-sodium veggie stock
- ½ cup cilantro, chopped
- Juice of 2 limes

Directions:
Heat up a pan with the oil over medium- high heat, add onion and garlic, stir and cook for 2 minutes. Add yellow and red bell pepper, stir, cook for 3 minutes more and transfer everything to your slow cooker. Add beans, cumin, water, stock and black pepper, stir, cover and cook on Low for 8 minutes. Add cilantro and lime juice, stir, ladle into bowls and serve.
Enjoy!

Nutrition: calories 200, fat 3, fiber 6, carbs 16, protein 8

Beet Soup

Preparation time: 10 minutes
Cooking time: 7 hours
Servings: 6

Ingredients:

- 1 and ¼ pounds beets, peeled and cut into wedges
- 2 tablespoons olive oil
- 1 red onion, chopped
- 2 garlic cloves, minced
- 1 apple, peeled, cored and sliced
- 4 and ½ cups low-sodium veggie stock
- 2 tablespoons apple cider vinegar
- 1 tablespoon stevia
- A pinch of black pepper

Directions:
Heat up a pan with the oil over medium- high heat, add the onion and the garlic stir, cook for 2-3 minutes and transfer to your slow cooker. Add beets, apple, stock, vinegar, stevia and black pepper, cover and cook on Low for 7 hours. Puree the soup using an immersion blender, ladle soup into bowls and serve.
Enjoy!

Nutrition: calories 132, fat 3, fiber 6, carbs 10, protein 5

Delicious Tomato Cream

Preparation time: 10 minutes
Cooking time: 4 hours
Servings: 8

Ingredients:

- 56 ounces tomatoes, chopped
- 1 small yellow onion, chopped
- 2 cups low-sodium veggie stock
- 1 teaspoon thyme, dried
- 1 teaspoon oregano, dried
- ½ teaspoon garlic powder
- A pinch of black pepper
- 1 bay leaf
- 4 tablespoon non-fat butter
- 1 cup fat-free milk

Directions:
In your slow cooker, combine the tomatoes with the onion, stock, thyme, oregano, garlic powder, black pepper, bay leaf, butter and milk, stir, cover and cook on High for 4 hours. Discard the bay leaf, puree the soup in batches in your blender, ladle into bowls and serve.
Enjoy!

Nutrition: calories 214, fat 4, fiber 8, carbs 16, protein 6

Rich Lentils Soup

Preparation time: 10 minutes
Cooking time: 6 hours
Servings: 6

Ingredients:
- 1 yellow onion, chopped
- 6 carrots, chopped
- 4 garlic cloves, minced
- 1 yellow bell pepper, chopped
- A pinch of cayenne pepper
- 4 cups red lentils
- 4 cups low sodium chicken stock
- 4 cups water
- Zest of 1 lemon, grated
- Juice of 1 lemon
- 1 tablespoon rosemary, chopped

Directions:
In your slow cooker, mix the onion with the carrots, garlic, bell pepper, cayenne, lentils, stock and water, stir, cover and cook on Low for 6 hours. Add lemon zest, lemon juice and rosemary, stir, ladle into bowls and serve.
Enjoy!

Nutrition: calories 261, fat 4, fiber 7, carbs 16, protein 10

Broccoli and Cauliflower Soup

Preparation time: 10 minutes
Cooking time: 8 hours
Servings: 4

Ingredients:
- 3 cups broccoli florets
- 2 cups cauliflower florets
- 2 garlic cloves, minced
- ½ cup shallots, chopped
- 1 carrot, chopped
- 3 and ½ cups low sodium veggie stock
- A pinch of black pepper
- 1 cup fat-free milk
- 6 ounce low-fat cheddar cheese, shredded
- 1 cup non-fat Greek yogurt

Directions:
In your slow cooker, mix the broccoli with cauliflower, garlic, shallots, carrot, stock and black pepper, cover and cook on Low for 8 hours. Transfer the soup to a blender, add milk and cheese and pulse well. Add the yogurt, pulse again, ladle into bowls and serve.
Enjoy!

Nutrition: calories 218, fat 11, fiber 7, carbs 15, protein 12

Butternut Squash Cream

Preparation time: 10 minutes
Cooking time: 4 hours
Servings: 6

Ingredients:
- 2 cups low sodium veggie stock
- 2 garlic cloves, minced
- 1 carrot, sliced
- 1 green apple, cored, peeled and chopped
- 1 medium butternut squash, peeled, deseeded and chopped
- 1 yellow onion, chopped
- 1 sage spring
- A pinch of black pepper
- A pinch of cayenne pepper
- A pinch of cinnamon powder
- A pinch of nutmeg, ground
- ½ cup coconut milk

Directions:
In your slow cooker, mix the stock with garlic, carrot, apple, squash, onion, sage, black pepper, cayenne, nutmeg and cinnamon, cover and cook on High for 4 hours. Add coconut milk, discard sage, blend the soup using an immersion blender, ladle into bowls and serve.
Enjoy!

Nutrition: calories 211, fat 3, fiber 5, carbs 15, protein 4

Chickpeas Mix

Preparation time: 10 minutes
Cooking time: 4 hours and 5 minutes
Servings: 6

Ingredients:
- 1 yellow onion, chopped
- 1 tablespoon ginger, grated
- 1 tablespoon olive oil
- 4 garlic cloves, minced
- A pinch of black pepper
- 2 red Thai chilies, chopped
- ½ teaspoon turmeric powder
- 2 tablespoons garam masala
- 4 ounces no-salt-added tomato paste
- 2 cups low sodium veggie stock
- 6 ounces canned chickpeas, drained and rinsed
- 2 tablespoons parsley, chopped

Directions:
Heat up a pan with the oil over medium- high heat, add ginger, onions, garlic, pepper, Thai chilies, garam masala and turmeric, stir, cook for 5-6 minutes more and transfer everything to your slow cooker. Add stock, chickpeas and tomato paste, stir, cover and cook on Low for 4 hours. Add parsley, stir, divide into bowls and serve.
Enjoy!

Nutrition: calories 211, fat 7, fiber 4, carbs 12, protein 7

Navy Beans Stew

Preparation time: 10 minutes
Cooking time: 12 hours
Servings: 6

Ingredients:
- 1 pound navy beans, soaked overnight and drained
- 1 cup maple syrup
- 1 cup no-salt tomato sauce
- 4 tablespoons stevia
- 1 cup water
- ¼ cup no-salt-added tomato paste
- ¼ cup mustard
- ¼ cup olive oil
- ¼ cup apple cider vinegar

Directions:
In your slow cooker, mix beans with maple syrup, tomato sauce, stevia, water, tomato paste, mustard, oil and vinegar, stir, cover, cook on Low for 12 hours, divide into bowls and serve. Enjoy!

Nutrition: calories 233, fat 7, fiber 12, carbs 15, protein 6

Potatoes Stew

Preparation time: 10 minutes
Cooking time: 3 hours
Servings: 4

Ingredients:
- 1 pound gold potatoes, peeled and cubed
- 1 small onion, chopped
- 2 tablespoons water
- 1 tablespoon olive oil
- ½ teaspoon cumin, ground
- ½ teaspoon coriander, ground
- ½ teaspoon garam masala
- ½ teaspoon chili powder
- 1 pound spinach, torn
- Black pepper to the taste

Directions:
In your slow cooker, mix potatoes with onion, water, oil, cumin, coriander, garam masala, chili, spinach and black pepper, stir, cover, cook on High for 3 hours, divide into bowls and serve. Enjoy!

Nutrition: calories 203, fat 4, fiber 7, carbs 12, protein 4

Easy Navy Beans Soup

Preparation time: 10 minutes
Cooking time: 4 hours
Servings: 6

Ingredients:
- 1 pounds navy beans, dried
- 1 yellow onion, chopped
- 2 quarts low-sodium veggie stock
- Black pepper to the taste
- 2 gold potatoes, cubed
- 1 pound carrots, sliced
- 1 cup sun-dried tomatoes, chopped
- 2 teaspoons dill, chopped
- 4 tablespoons parsley, chopped

Directions:
In your slow cooker, mix beans with onion, stock, pepper, potatoes, carrots, tomatoes, dill and parsley, stir, cover, cook on High for 4 hours, ladle into bowls and serve.
Enjoy!

Nutrition: calories 221, fat 4, fiber 8, carbs 15, protein 4

Black Beans and Mango Mix

Preparation time: 10 minutes
Cooking time: 6 hours and 15 minutes
Servings: 6

Ingredients:
- 1 yellow onion, chopped
- 1 tablespoon olive oil
- 1 red bell pepper, chopped
- 1 jalapeno, chopped
- 2 garlic cloves, minced
- 2 mangoes, peeled, cored and chopped
- 1 teaspoon ginger, grated
- ½ teaspoon cumin, ground
- ½ teaspoon allspice, ground
- ½ teaspoon oregano, dried
- 30 ounces canned black beans, no-salt-added, drained and rinsed
- ½ teaspoon stevia
- 1 cup water
- A pinch of black pepper
- 2 cups brown rice, cooked

Directions:
Heat up a pan with the oil over medium- high heat, add onion, garlic, ginger and jalapeno, stir, cook for 3 minutes and transfer to your slow cooker. Add red bell pepper, cumin, allspice, oregano, black beans, stevia, water and pepper, stir, cover and cook on Low for 6 hours. Add rice and mangoes, stir, cover, cook on Low for 10 minutes more, divide between plates and serve.
Enjoy!

Nutrition: calories 260, fat 6, fiber 13, carbs 8, protein 11

Spinach Soup

Preparation time: 10 minutes
Cooking time: 10 hours
Servings: 8

Ingredients:
- 10 ounces baby spinach
- 2 celery ribs, chopped
- 2 carrots, chopped
- 1 garlic clove, minced
- 1 yellow onion, chopped
- 4 cups veggie stock
- 28 ounces canned tomatoes, no-salt-added and chopped
- 2 bay leaves
- 1 teaspoon oregano, dried
- 1 tablespoon cilantro, chopped
- ½ teaspoon red pepper flakes, crushed

Directions:
In your slow cooker, mix spinach with celery, carrots, garlic, onion, stock, tomatoes, bay leaves, oregano, cilantro, red pepper flakes, stir, cover, cook on Low for 10 hours, ladle into bowls and serve.
Enjoy!

Nutrition: calories 190, fat 4, fiber 4, carbs 11, protein 6

Asian Salmon

Preparation time: 10 minutes
Cooking time: 3 hours
Servings: 2

Ingredients:
- 2 medium salmon fillets, boneless
- Black pepper to the taste
- 2 tablespoons low sodium soy sauce
- 2 tablespoons maple syrup
- 16 ounces mixed broccoli and cauliflower florets
- 2 tablespoons lemon juice
- 1 teaspoon sesame seeds

Directions:
Put the cauliflower and broccoli florets in your slow cooker and top with the salmon. In a bowl, mix maple syrup with soy sauce and lemon juice, whisk, and pour over the salmon mix, season with black pepper to the taste, sprinkle sesame seeds on top and cook on Low for 3 hours. Divide everything between plates and serve.
Enjoy!

Nutrition: calories 230, fat 4, fiber 2, carbs 13, protein 6

Seafood Stew

Preparation time: 10 minutes
Cooking time: 3 hours and 30 minutes
Servings: 6

Ingredients:
- 3 garlic cloves, minced
- 28 ounces canned tomatoes, no-salt-added and crushed
- 1 pound sweet potatoes, peeled and cubed
- 4 cups low sodium veggie stock
- 1 small yellow onion, chopped
- 1 teaspoon cilantro, dried
- 1 teaspoon thyme, dried
- 1 teaspoon basil, dried
- Black pepper to the taste
- ¼ teaspoon red pepper flakes
- A pinch of cayenne pepper
- 1 pound scallops
- 1 pound shrimp, peeled and deveined

Directions:
Put tomatoes in your slow cooker; add garlic, sweet potatoes, stock, onion, cilantro, thyme, basil, pepper, cayenne and pepper flakes, stir, cover and cook on High for 3 hours. Add scallops and shrimp, stir gently, cover, cook on High for 30 minutes more, divide into bowls and serve.
Enjoy!

Nutrition: calories 230, fat 3, fiber 2, carbs 14, protein 6

Slow Cooked Tuna

Preparation time: 10 minutes
Cooking time: 4 hours and 10 minutes
Servings: 2

Ingredients:
- ½ pound tuna loin, cubed
- 1 garlic clove, minced
- 4 jalapeno peppers, chopped
- 1 cup olive oil
- 3 red chili peppers, chopped
- 2 teaspoons black peppercorns, ground
- Black pepper to the taste

Directions:
Put the oil in your slow cooker; add chili peppers, jalapenos, peppercorns, pepper and garlic, whisk, cover and cook on Low for 4 hours. Add tuna, toss, cook on High for 10 minutes more, divide between plates and serve.
Enjoy!

Nutrition: calories 190, fat 4, fiber 3, carbs 10, protein 4

Herbed Salmon

Preparation time: 10 minutes
Cooking time: 2 hours and 30 minutes
Servings: 4

Ingredients:
- 2 garlic cloves, minced
- 4 salmon fillets, boneless and skin on
- 1 cup cilantro, chopped
- 3 tablespoons lime juice
- 1 tablespoon olive oil
- Black pepper to the taste

Directions:
Grease your slow cooker with the oil, place salmon fillets inside, add garlic, cilantro, lime juice and pepper, cover and cook on Low for 2 hours and 30 minutes. Divide salmon between plates, drizzle the cilantro sauce from the slow cooker all over and serve.
Enjoy!

Nutrition: calories 220, fat 3, fiber 2, carbs 14, protein 8

Coconut Clams

Preparation time: 10 minutes
Cooking time: 6 hours
Servings: 4

Ingredients:
- 21 ounces canned clams, no-salt-added, drained and chopped
- 1/3 cup coconut milk
- 4 eggs, whisked
- 2 tablespoons olive oil
- 1/3 cup green bell pepper, chopped
- ½ cup yellow onion, chopped
- Black pepper to the taste

Directions:
Put clams in your slow cooker; add milk, eggs, oil, onion, bell pepper and black pepper, toss, cover, cook on Low for 6 hours, divide into bowls and serve.
Enjoy!

Nutrition: calories 200, fat 4, fiber 2, carbs 12, protein 7

Creamy Seafood and Veggies Soup

Preparation time: 10 minutes
Cooking time: 3 hours
Servings: 12

Ingredients:

- 10 ounces coconut cream
- 2 cups low-sodium veggie stock
- 2 cups no-salt-added tomato sauce
- 12 ounces canned crab meat, no-salt-added and drained
- 1 and ½ cups water
- 1 and ½ pounds jumbo shrimp, peeled and deveined
- 1 yellow onion, chopped
- 1 cup carrots, chopped
- 4 tilapia fillets, skinless, boneless and cubed
- 2 celery stalks, chopped
- 3 kale stalks, chopped
- 1 bay leaf
- 2 garlic cloves, minced
- ½ teaspoon cloves, ground
- 1 teaspoon rosemary, dried
- 1 teaspoon thyme, dried

Directions:
In your slow cooker, mix coconut cream with stock, tomato sauce and water and stir. Add shrimp, fish, onion, carrots, celery, kale, garlic, bay leaf, cloves, thyme and rosemary, cover, cook on Low for 3 hours, stir, ladle into bowls and serve.
Enjoy!

Nutrition: calories 220, fat 3, fiber 3, carbs 8, protein 7

Seafood Gumbo

Preparation time: 10 minutes
Cooking time: 6 hours
Servings: 4

Ingredients:

- 1 pound shrimp, peeled and deveined
- 2 pounds mussels, cleaned and debearded
- 28 ounces canned clams, no-salt-added and drained
- 1 yellow onion, chopped
- 10 ounces canned tomato paste, no-salt-added

Directions:
In your slow cooker, mix shrimp with mussels, clams, onion and tomato paste, stir, cover, cook on Low for 6 hours, divide into bowls and serve.
Enjoy!

Nutrition: calories 200, fat 3, fiber 2, carbs 7, protein 5

Lemon and Spinach Trout

Preparation time: 10 minutes
Cooking time: 2 hours
Servings: 4

Ingredients:
- 2 lemons, sliced
- ¼ cup low sodium chicken stock
- Black pepper to the taste
- 2 tablespoons dill, chopped
- 12 ounces spinach
- 4 medium trout

Directions:
Put the stock in your slow cooker, add the fish inside Season with black pepper to the taste, top with lemon slices, dill and spinach, cover, and cook on High for 2 hours. Divide fish, lemon and spinach between plates and serve.
Enjoy!

Nutrition: calories 240, fat 5, fiber 4, carbs 9, protein 14

Mexican Chicken

Preparation time: 10 minutes
Cooking time: 7 hours
Servings: 4

Ingredients:
- 4 chicken breasts, skinless and boneless
- ½ cup water
- 16 ounces chunky salsa
- 1 and ½ tablespoons parsley, chopped
- 1 teaspoon garlic powder
- ½ tablespoon cilantro, chopped
- 1 teaspoon onion powder
- ½ tablespoons oregano, dried
- ½ teaspoon sweet paprika
- 1 teaspoon chili powder
- ½ teaspoon cumin, ground
- Black pepper to the taste

Directions:
Put the water in your slow cooker, add chicken breasts, salsa, parsley, garlic powder, cilantro, onion powder, oregano, paprika, chili powder, cumin and black pepper to the taste, toss, cover and cook on Low for 7 hours. Divide the whole mix between plates and serve.
Enjoy!

Nutrition: calories 200, fat 4, fiber 2, carbs 12, protein 9

Chicken Breast Stew

Preparation time: 10 minutes
Cooking time: 8 hours
Servings: 4

Ingredients:
- 1 yellow onion, chopped
- 2 pounds chicken breasts, skinless and boneless
- 4 ounces canned jalapenos, drained and chopped
- 1 green bell pepper, chopped
- 4 ounces canned green chilies, drained and chopped
- 7 ounces tomato sauce
- 14 ounces canned tomatoes, chopped
- 2 tablespoons coconut oil, melted
- 3 garlic cloves, minced
- 1 tablespoon chili powder
- 1 tablespoon cumin, ground
- 2 teaspoons oregano, dried
- A bunch of cilantro, chopped
- Black pepper to the taste
- 1 avocado, pitted, peeled and sliced

Directions:
Grease the slow cooker with the melted oil, add onion, chicken, jalapenos, bell pepper, green chilies, tomato sauce, tomatoes, garlic, chili powder, cumin, oregano and black pepper, stir, cover and cook on Low for 8 hours. Add cilantro, shred chicken breasts using 2 forks, stir the stew, divide into bowls and top with avocado slices.
Enjoy!

Nutrition: calories 205, fat 4, fiber 5, carbs 9, protein 11

Turkey Breast and Sweet Potato Mix

Preparation time: 10 minutes
Cooking time: 8 hours
Servings: 4

Ingredients:
- 3 pounds turkey breast, bone in
- 3 sweet potatoes, cut into wedges
- 1 cup dried cherries, pitted
- 2 white onions, cut into wedges
- 1/3 cup water
- 1 teaspoon onion powder
- 1 teaspoon garlic powder
- 1 teaspoon parsley flakes
- 1 teaspoon thyme, dried
- 1 teaspoon sage, dried
- 1 teaspoon paprika, dried
- Black pepper to the taste

Directions:
Put the turkey breast in your slow cooker, add sweet potatoes, cherries, onions, water, parsley, garlic and onion powder, thyme, sage, paprika and pepper, toss, cover and cook on Low for 8 hours. Discard bone from turkey breast, slice meat and divide between plates. Serve with the veggies and the cherries on the side.
Enjoy!

Nutrition: calories 220, fat 5, fiber 4, carbs 8, protein 15

Italian Chicken

Preparation time: 10 minutes
Cooking time: 5 hours
Servings: 4

Ingredients:
- 4 chicken breasts, skinless and boneless
- 6 Italian sausages, sliced
- 5 garlic cloves, minced
- 1 white onion, chopped
- 1 teaspoon Italian seasoning
- A drizzle of olive oil
- 1 teaspoon garlic powder
- 29 ounces canned tomatoes, chopped
- 15 ounces tomato sauce, no-salt-added
- 1 cup water
- ½ cup balsamic vinegar

Directions:
Put chicken and sausage slices in your slow cooker, add garlic, onion, Italian seasoning, the oil, tomatoes, tomato sauce, garlic powder, water and the vinegar, cover and cook on High for 5 hours. Stir chicken and sausage mix, divide between plates and serve.
Enjoy!

Nutrition: calories 237, fat 4, fiber 3, carbs 12, protein 13

Chicken Breast and Cinnamon Veggie Mix

Preparation time: 10 minutes
Cooking time: 6 hours
Servings: 4

Ingredients:
- 2 red bell peppers, chopped
- 2 pounds chicken breasts, skinless and boneless
- 4 garlic cloves, minced
- 1 yellow onion, chopped
- 2 teaspoons paprika
- 1 cup low sodium chicken stock
- 2 teaspoons cinnamon powder
- ¼ teaspoon nutmeg, ground

Directions:
In a bowl, mix bell peppers with chicken breasts, garlic, onion, paprika, cinnamon and nutmeg, toss to coat, transfer everything to your slow cooker, add stock, cover, cook on Low for 6 hours, divide everything between plates and serve.
Enjoy!

Nutrition: calories 200, fat 3, fiber 5, carbs 13, protein 8

Mexican Pork Mix

Preparation time: 10 minutes
Cooking time: 8 hours and 3 minutes
Servings: 6

Ingredients:
- 1 yellow onion, chopped
- 2 tablespoons sweet paprika
- 15 ounces canned tomatoes, no-salt-added, roasted and chopped
- 1 teaspoon cumin, ground
- 1 teaspoon olive oil
- Black pepper to the taste
- A pinch of nutmeg, ground
- 5 pounds pork roast, trimmed
- Juice of 1 lemon
- ¼ cup apple cider vinegar

Directions:
Heat up a pan with the oil over medium- high heat, add onions, stir, brown them for 2-3 minutes, transfer them to your slow cooker, add paprika, tomato, cumin, nutmeg, lemon juice, vinegar, black pepper and pork, toss to coat, cover and cook on Low for 8 hours. Slice roast, divide between plates and serve with tomatoes and onions mix on the side.
Enjoy!

Nutrition: calories 250, fat 5, fiber 2, carbs 8, protein 15

Maple Pork Tenderloin

Preparation time: 10 minutes
Cooking time: 8 hours
Servings: 4

Ingredients:
- A pinch of nutmeg, ground
- 2 pounds pork tenderloin, trimmed
- 4 apples, cored and sliced
- 2 tablespoons maple syrup

Directions:
Place half of the apples in your slow cooker, sprinkle the nutmeg over them, add pork tenderloin, top with the rest of the apples, drizzle the maple syrup, cover and cook on Low for 8 hours. Slice pork tenderloin, divide between plates and serve with apple slices and cooking juices on top.
Enjoy!

Nutrition: calories 240, fat 4, fiber 5, carbs 14, protein 14

Pork and Cabbage Stew

Preparation time: 10 minutes
Cooking time: 8 hours and 10 minutes
Servings: 6

Ingredients:
- 1 tablespoon olive oil
- 2 pounds pork loin, cubed
- 3 garlic cloves, minced
- 6 baby carrots, halved
- 2 onions, chopped
- Black pepper to the taste
- 1 cabbage head, shredded
- 3 cups veggie stock
- 28 ounces canned tomatoes, no-salt-added, drained and chopped
- 3 big sweet potatoes, cubed

Directions:
Heat up a pan with the oil over medium- high heat, add meat, brown for a few minutes on each side, transfer to your slow cooker, add black pepper, carrots, garlic, onion, potatoes, cabbage, stock and tomatoes, stir well, cover, cook on Low for 8 hours, divide the stew into bowls and serve right away.
Enjoy!

Nutrition: calories 270, fat 5, fiber 4, carbs 14, protein 7

Greek Pork

Preparation time: 1 day
Cooking time: 8 hours
Servings: 6

Ingredients:
- 3 pounds pork shoulder, boneless
- ¼ cup olive oil
- 2 teaspoons oregano, dried
- ¼ cup lemon juice
- 2 teaspoons mustard
- 2 teaspoons mint
- 6 garlic cloves, minced
- Black pepper to the taste

Directions:
In a bowl, mix oil with lemon juice, oregano, mint, mustard, garlic and pepper, whisk, rub the meat with the marinade, cover and keep in the fridge for 1 day. Transfer to your slow cooker along with the marinade, cover, cook on Low for 8 hours, slice the roast and serve.
Enjoy!

Nutrition: calories 260, fat 4, fiber 6, carbs 14, protein 8

Roast and Veggies

Preparation time: 10 minutes
Cooking time: 4 hours
Servings: 6

Ingredients:

- 1 pound sweet potatoes, chopped
- 3 and ½ pounds pork roast, trimmed
- 8 medium carrots, chopped
- 15 ounces canned tomatoes, no-salt-added and chopped
- 1 yellow onion, chopped
- Zest of 1 lemon, grated
- Juice of 1 lemon
- 4 garlic cloves, minced
- Black pepper to the taste
- ½ cup kalamata olives, pitted

Directions:
Put potatoes in your slow cooker, carrots, tomatoes, onions, lemon juice and zest, pork, black pepper and garlic, stir, cover and cook on High for 4 hours. Transfer meat to a cutting board, slice it and divide between plates. Transfer the veggies to a bowl, mash, mix them with olives, and add next to the meat.
Enjoy!

Nutrition: calories 250, fat 4, fiber 3, carbs 15, protein 13

Pork Roast Soup

Preparation time: 10 minutes
Cooking time: 7 hours
Servings: 4

Ingredients:

- 2 pounds pork roast
- 6 red onions, sliced
- 2 quarts low sodium veggie stock
- 4 thyme springs
- ½ cup sherry vinegar
- 1 bay leaf
- A pinch of black pepper
- 2 tablespoons olive oil

Directions:
In your slow cooker, mix the roast with stock, bay leaf and thyme, cover, cook on High for 6 hours, transfer roast to a cutting board, shred and transfer to a bowl. Heat up a large pot with the oil over medium-high heat, add onions, stir, cook them for 5 minutes and transfer to your slow cooker, Add vinegar, some pepper and return the meat, stir, cover, cook for 45 minutes more, ladle into bowls and serve.
Enjoy!

Nutrition: calories 332, fat 7, fiber 7, carbs 12, protein 14

Coconut Salmon Soup

Preparation time: 10 minutes
Cooking time: 4 hours
Servings: 6

Ingredients:
- 2 tablespoons olive oil
- 4 leeks, sliced
- 3 garlic cloves, minced
- 6 cups low sodium chicken stock
- 2 teaspoons thyme, dried
- 1 pounds salmon, skinless, boneless and cubed
- 1 and ¼ cup coconut milk
- A pinch of black pepper

Directions:
Heat up a pan with the oil over medium-high heat, add garlic and leeks, stir, brown for a few minutes, transfer them to your slow cooker, add stock, thyme and pepper, cover and cook on Low for 3 hours. Add coconut milk and salmon, cover, cook on Low for 1 hour, ladle into bowls and serve.
Enjoy!

Nutrition: calories 232, fat 4, fiber 7, carbs 9, protein11

Ground Pork and Veggies Soup

Preparation time: 10 minutes
Cooking time: 6 hours and 10 minutes
Servings: 4

Ingredients:
- 1 pound pork, ground
- 2 zucchinis, chopped
- 1 carrot, chopped
- 1 yellow onion, chopped
- 1 celery stalk, chopped
- ½ cup low sodium veggie stock
- 3 cups water
- A pinch of black pepper
- 29 ounces canned tomatoes, no-salt-added and chopped
- 1 tablespoon garlic, minced
- ½ teaspoon oregano, dried
- ½ teaspoon basil, dried

Directions:
Heat up a pan over medium-high heat, add meat, brown for a few minutes, transfer to your slow cooker, add water, zucchinis, carrot, onion, celery, stock, pepper, tomatoes, garlic, oregano and basil, stir, cover, cook on Low for 6 hours, ladle into bowls and serve.
Enjoy!

Nutrition: calories 231, fat 6, fiber 7, carbs 14, protein 12

Greek Cod Mix

Preparation time: 10 minutes
Cooking time: 2 hours
Servings: 4

Ingredients:
- 4 cod fillets, boneless and skinless
- 1 cup black olives, pitted and chopped
- 1 tablespoon olive oil
- 1 garlic clove, minced
- ½ cup low sodium veggie stock
- A pinch of black pepper
- 1 pound cherry tomatoes, halved
- A pinch of thyme, dried

Directions:
In your slow cooker, mix cod with black olives, oil, garlic, stock, pepper, cherry tomatoes and thyme, cover, cook on High for 2 hours, divide everything between plates and serve.
Enjoy!

Nutrition: calories 220, fat 3, fiber 4, carbs 13, protein 11

Creamy Fish Curry

Preparation time: 10 minutes
Cooking time: 2 hours
Servings: 6

Ingredients:
- 6 cod fillets, skinless, boneless and cubed
- 1 tomato, chopped
- 14 ounces coconut milk, unsweetened
- 2 yellow onions, sliced
- 2 green bell peppers, chopped
- 2 garlic cloves, minced
- ½ teaspoon turmeric powder
- 6 curry leaves
- A pinch of black pepper
- 2 teaspoons cumin, ground
- 2 tablespoons lemon juice
- 1 tablespoons coriander, ground
- 1 tablespoon ginger, grated

Directions:
In your slow cooker, mix fish with tomato, coconut milk, onions, green bell peppers, garlic, curry leaves, turmeric, pepper, cumin, lemon juice, coriander and ginger, toss, cover, cook on High for 2 hours, divide into bowls and serve.
Enjoy!

Nutrition: calories 221, fat 7, fiber 3, carbs 11, protein 13

Hot Mackerel

Preparation time: 10 minutes
Cooking time: 2 hours and 30 minutes
Servings: 4

Ingredients:
- 18 ounces mackerel, skinless, boneless and cut into pieces
- 3 garlic cloves, minced
- 8 shallots, chopped
- 1 teaspoon turmeric powder
- 1 tablespoon chili paste
- 2 lemongrass sticks, halved
- 1 ginger slice, grated
- 3 and ½ ounces water
- 5 tablespoons olive oil
- 1 and 1/3 tablespoons tamarind paste

Directions:
In your blender, mix garlic with shallots, chili paste and turmeric, blend well and add to slow cooker. Add fish, oil, ginger, lemongrass, tamarind and water, stir, cover, cook on Low for 2 hours and 30 minutes, divide between plates and serve.
Enjoy!

Nutrition: calories 212, fat 8, fiber 4, carbs 12, protein 12

Mussels Mix

Preparation time: 10 minutes
Cooking time: 2 hours
Servings: 4

Ingredients:
- 2 pounds mussels, scrubbed
- 2 tablespoons olive oil
- 1 yellow onion, chopped
- 1 teaspoon parsley, dried
- ½ teaspoon red pepper flakes, crushed
- 2 teaspoons garlic, minced
- 14 ounces canned tomatoes, no-salt-added and chopped
- ½ cup low sodium chicken stock

Directions:
In your slow cooker, mix mussels with oil, onion parsley, pepper flakes, garlic, tomatoes and stock, stir, cover, cook on High for 2 hours, divide into bowls and serve.
Enjoy!

Nutrition: calories 200, fat 2, fiber 3, carbs 13, protein 6

Turkey Wings and Veggies

Preparation time: 10 minutes
Cooking time: 8 hours
Servings: 4

Ingredients:
- 4 turkey wings
- 1 yellow onion, chopped
- 1 carrot, chopped
- 3 garlic cloves, minced
- 1 celery stalk, chopped
- 1 cup low sodium chicken stock
- Black pepper to the taste
- 2 tablespoons olive oil
- 1 teaspoon rosemary, dried
- A pinch of sage, dried
- A pinch of thyme, dried

Directions:
In your slow cooker, mix turkey wings with the onion, carrot, garlic, celery, stock, black pepper, oil, rosemary, sage and thyme, toss, cover, cook on Low for 8 hours, divide between plates and serve.
Enjoy!

Nutrition: calories 223, fat 5, fiber 7, carbs 15, protein 14

Citrus Turkey Mix

Preparation time: 10 minutes
Cooking time: 8 hours
Servings: 4

Ingredients:
- 4 turkey wings
- 2 tablespoons olive oil
- 1 and ½ cups cranberries, dried
- Black pepper to the taste
- 1 yellow onion, chopped
- 1 cup walnuts, chopped
- 1 cup orange juice
- 1 bunch thyme, chopped

Directions:
Grease the slow cooker with the oil, add turkey wings, cranberries, pepper, onion, walnuts, orange juice and thyme, cover, cook on Low for 8 hours, divide everything between plates and serve.
Enjoy!

Nutrition: calories 270, fat 12, fiber 4, carbs 14, protein 5

Dash Diet Slow Cooker Side Dish Recipes

Broccoli Mix

Preparation time: 10 minutes
Cooking time: 3 hours
Servings: 10

Ingredients:
- 6 cups broccoli florets
- 10 ounces tomato sauce, sodium-free
- 1 and ½ cups low-fat cheddar cheese, shredded
- ½ teaspoon Worcestershire sauce
- ¼ cup yellow onion, chopped
- A pinch of black pepper
- 2 tablespoons olive oil

Directions:
Grease your slow cooker with the oil, add broccoli, tomato sauce, Worcestershire sauce, onion and black pepper, cover and cook on High for 2 hours and 30 minutes. Sprinkle the cheese all over, cover, cook on High for 30 minutes more, divide between plates and serve as a side dish. Enjoy!

Nutrition: calories 160, fat 6, fiber 4, carbs 11, protein 6

Tasty Bean Side Dish

Preparation time: 10 minutes
Cooking time: 5 hours
Servings: 10

Ingredients:
- 1 and ½ cups tomato sauce, salt-free
- 1 yellow onion, chopped
- 2 celery ribs, chopped
- 1 sweet red pepper, chopped
- 1 green bell pepper, chopped
- ½ cup water
- 2 bay leaves
- 1 teaspoon ground mustard
- 1 tablespoon cider vinegar
- 16 ounces canned kidney beans, no-salt-added, drained and rinsed
- 16 ounces canned black-eyed peas, no-salt-added, drained and rinsed
- 15 ounces corn
- 15 ounces canned lima beans, no-salt-added, drained and rinsed
- 15 ounces canned black beans, no-salt-added, drained and rinsed

Directions:
In your slow cooker, mix the tomato sauce with the onion, celery, red pepper, green bell pepper, water, bay leaves, mustard, vinegar, kidney beans, black-eyed peas, corn, lima beans and black beans, cover and cook on Low for 5 hours. Discard bay leaves, divide the whole mix between plates and serve.
Enjoy!

Nutrition: calories 211, fat 4, fiber 8, carbs 20, protein 7

Easy Green Beans

Preparation time: 10 minutes
Cooking time: 2 hours
Servings: 12

Ingredients:
- 16 ounces green beans
- 3 tablespoons olive oil
- ½ cup coconut sugar
- 1 teaspoon low-sodium soy sauce
- ½ teaspoon garlic powder

Directions:
In your slow cooker, mix the green beans with the oil, sugar, soy sauce and garlic powder, cover and cook on Low for 2 hours. Toss the beans, divide them between plates and serve as a side dish.
Enjoy!

Nutrition: calories 142, fat 7, fiber 4, carbs 15, protein 3

Creamy Corn

Preparation time: 10 minutes
Cooking time: 4 hours
Servings: 12

Ingredients:
- 10 cups corn
- 20 ounces fat-free cream cheese
- ½ cup fat-free milk
- ½ cup low-fat butter
- A pinch of black pepper
- 2 tablespoons green onions, chopped

Directions:
In your slow cooker, mix the corn with cream cheese, milk, butter, black pepper and onions, toss, cover and cook on Low for 4 hours. Toss one more time, divide between plates and serve as a side dish.
Enjoy!

Nutrition: calories 256, fat 11, fiber 2, carbs 17, protein 5

Classic Peas and Carrots

Preparation time: 10 minutes
Cooking time: 5 hours
Servings: 12

Ingredients:
- 1 pound carrots, sliced
- ¼ cup water
- 1 yellow onion, chopped
- 2 tablespoons olive oil
- ¼ cup honey
- 4 garlic cloves, minced
- 1 teaspoon marjoram, dried
- A pinch of white pepper
- 16 ounces peas

Directions:
In your slow cooker, mix the carrots with water, onion, oil, honey, garlic, marjoram, white pepper and peas, toss, cover and cook on High for 5 hours. Divide between plates and serve as a side dish.
Enjoy!

Nutrition: calories 107, fat 3, fiber 3, carbs 14, protein 4

Mushroom Pilaf

Preparation time: 10 minutes
Cooking time: 3 hours
Servings: 6

Ingredients:
- 1 cup wild rice
- 2 garlic cloves, minced
- 6 green onions, chopped
- 2 tablespoons olive oil
- ½ pound baby Bella mushrooms
- 2 cups water

Directions:
In your slow cooker, mix the rice with garlic, onions, oil, mushrooms and water, toss, cover and cook on Low for 3 hours. Stir the pilaf one more time, divide between plates and serve.
Enjoy!

Nutrition: calories 210, fat 7, fiber 1, carbs 16, protein 4

Butternut Mix

Preparation time: 10 minutes
Cooking time: 4 hours
Servings: 8

Ingredients:
- 1 cup carrots, chopped
- 1 tablespoon olive oil
- 1 yellow onion, chopped
- ½ teaspoon stevia
- 1 garlic clove, minced
- ½ teaspoon curry powder
- ½ teaspoon cinnamon powder
- ¼ teaspoon ginger, grated
- 1 butternut squash, cubed
- 2 and ½ cups low-sodium veggie stock
- ½ cup basmati rice
- ¾ cup coconut milk

Directions:
Heat up a pan with the oil over medium- high heat, add the oil, onion, garlic, stevia, carrots, curry powder, cinnamon and ginger, stir, cook for 5 minutes and transfer to your slow cooker. Add squash, stock and coconut milk, stir, cover and cook on Low for 4 hours. Divide the butternut mix between plates and serve as a side dish.
Enjoy!

Nutrition: calories 200, fat 4, fiber 4, carbs 17, protein 3

Sausage Side Dish

Preparation time: 10 minutes
Cooking time: 2 hours
Servings: 12

Ingredients:
- 1 pound no-sugar, pork sausage, chopped
- 2 tablespoons olive oil
- ½ pound mushrooms, chopped
- 6 celery ribs, chopped
- 2 yellow onions, chopped
- 2 garlic cloves, minced
- 1 tablespoon sage, dried
- 1 cup low-sodium veggie stock
- 1 cup cranberries, dried
- ½ cup sunflower seeds, peeled
- 1 whole wheat bread loaf, cubed

Directions:
Heat up a pan with the oil over medium- high heat, add pork, stir and brown for a few minutes. Add mushrooms, onion, celery, garlic and sage, stir, cook for a few more minutes and transfer to your slow cooker. Add stock, cranberries, sunflower seeds and the bread cubes, cover and cook on High for 2 hours. Stir the whole mix, divide between plates and serve as a side dish.
Enjoy!

Nutrition: calories 200, fat 3, fiber 6, carbs 13, protein 4

Easy Potatoes Mix

Preparation time: 10 minutes
Cooking time: 6 hours
Servings: 8

Ingredients:
- 16 baby red potatoes, halved
- 1 carrot, sliced
- 1 celery rib, chopped
- ¼ cup yellow onion, chopped
- 2 cups low-sodium chicken stock
- 1 tablespoon parsley, chopped
- A pinch of black pepper
- 1 garlic clove minced
- 2 tablespoons olive oil

Directions:
In your slow cooker, mix the potatoes with the carrot, celery, onion, stock, parsley, garlic, oil and black pepper, toss, cover and cook on Low for 6 hours. Divide between plates and serve as a side dish.
Enjoy!

Nutrition: calories 114, fat 3, fiber 3, carbs 18, protein 4

Black-Eyed Peas Mix

Preparation time: 10 minutes
Cooking time: 5 hours
Servings: 12

Ingredients:
- 17 ounces black-eyed peas
- ½ cup sausage, chopped
- 1 yellow onion, chopped
- 1 sweet red pepper, chopped
- 1 jalapeno, chopped
- 2 garlic cloves minced
- ½ teaspoon cumin, ground
- A pinch of black pepper
- 6 cups water
- 2 tablespoons cilantro, chopped

Directions:
In your slow cooker, mix the peas with the sausage, onion, red pepper, jalapeno, garlic, cumin, black pepper, water and cilantro, cover and cook on Low for 5 hours. Divide between plates and serve as a side dish.
Enjoy!

Nutrition: calories 170, fat 3, fiber 7, carbs 20, protein 13

Green Beans and Corn Mix

Preparation time: 10 minutes
Cooking time: 4 hours
Servings: 8

Ingredients:
- 15 ounces green beans
- 14 ounces corn
- 11 ounces cream of mushroom soup, low-fat and sodium-free
- 4 ounces mushrooms, sliced
- ½ cup almonds, chopped
- ½ cup low-fat cheddar cheese, shredded
- ½ cup low-fat sour cream

Directions:
In your slow cooker, mix the green beans with the corn, mushrooms soup, mushrooms, almonds, cheese and sour cream, toss, cover and cook on Low for 4 hours. Stir one more time, divide between plates and serve as a side dish.
Enjoy!

Nutrition: calories 211, fat 8, fiber 3, carbs 16, protein 4

Spiced Carrots

Preparation time: 10 minutes
Cooking time: 6 hours
Servings: 6

Ingredients:
- 2 pounds small carrots, peeled
- ½ cup low-fat butter, melted
- ½ cup canned peach, unsweetened
- 3 tablespoons stevia
- ½ teaspoon cinnamon powder
- 1 teaspoon vanilla extract
- A pinch of nutmeg, ground
- 2 tablespoons water
- 2 tablespoons cornstarch

Directions:
In your slow cooker, mix the carrots with the butter, peach, stevia, cinnamon, vanilla, nutmeg and cornstarch mixed with water, toss, cover and cook on Low for 6 hours. Toss the carrots one more time, divide between plates and serve as a side dish.
Enjoy!

Nutrition: calories 200, fat 12, fiber 4, carbs 20, protein 3

Squash and Grains Mix

Preparation time: 10 minutes
Cooking time: 4 hours
Servings: 12

Ingredients:
- 1 butternut squash, peeled and cubed
- 1 cup whole grain blend, uncooked
- 1 yellow onion, chopped
- 3 garlic cloves, minced
- ½ cup water
- 2 teaspoons thyme, chopped
- A pinch of black pepper
- 12 ounces low-sodium veggie stock
- 6 ounces baby spinach

Directions:
In your slow cooker, mix the squash with whole grain, onion, garlic, water, thyme, black pepper, stock and spinach, cover and cook on Low for 4 hours. Divide between plates and serve as a side dish.
Enjoy!

Nutrition: calories 100, fat 1, fiber 4, carbs 22, protein 3

Mushroom Mix

Preparation time: 10 minutes
Cooking time: 4 hours
Servings: 6

Ingredients:
- 1 pound mushrooms, halved
- 3 tablespoons olive oil
- 1 yellow onion, chopped
- 1 teaspoon Italian seasoning
- 1 cup tomato sauce, no-salt-added

Directions:
In your slow cooker, mix the mushrooms with the oil, onion, Italian seasoning and tomato sauce, toss, cover and cook on Low for 4 hours. Divide between plates and serve as a side dish.
Enjoy!

Nutrition: calories 100, fat 5, fiber 2, carbs 9, protein 4

Spinach and Rice

Preparation time: 10 minutes
Cooking time: 4 hours
Servings: 8

Ingredients:
- 2 tablespoons olive oil
- 1 yellow onion, chopped
- ¼ teaspoon thyme, dried
- 2 garlic cloves, minced
- 4 cups low-sodium chicken stock
- 20 ounces spinach, chopped
- 8 ounces fat-free cream cheese
- 2 cups wild rice
- 2 cups low-fat cheddar cheese, shredded
- ½ cup whole wheat bread, crumbled

Directions:
In your slow cooker, mix the oil with the onion, thyme, garlic, stock, spinach, cream cheese and rice, toss, cover and cook on Low for 4 hours. Add the cheese and the breadcrumbs cover the pot, leave it aside for a few minutes, divide between plates and serve as a side dish.
Enjoy!

Nutrition: calories 199, fat 2, fiber 6, carbs 9, protein 6

Creamy Mushrooms Mix

Preparation time: 10 minutes
Cooking time: 8 hours
Servings: 8

Ingredients:
- 1 and ½ pounds cremini mushrooms, halved
- 2 garlic cloves, minced
- 1 shallot, chopped
- ¼ cup low sodium chicken stock
- 2 tablespoons parsley, chopped
- ½ cup coconut cream
- 1 teaspoon cornstarch

Directions:
In your slow cooker, mix the mushrooms with garlic, shallot, stock and parsley, cover and cook on Low for 7 hours. Add coconut cream mixed with the cornstarch, cover, cook on Low for 1 more hour, divide between plates and serve as a side dish.
Enjoy!

Nutrition: calories 188, fat 3, fiber 8, carbs 17, protein 4

Ginger Beets

Preparation time: 10 minutes
Cooking time: 6 hours
Servings: 8

Ingredients:
- 6 beets, peeled and sliced
- 1 teaspoon orange peel, grated
- 2 tablespoons honey
- 1/3 cup orange juice
- 2 tablespoons white vinegar
- 2 tablespoons olive oil
- 1 tablespoon ginger, grated
- A pinch of black pepper

Directions:
In your slow cooker, mix the beets with the orange peel, orange juice, honey, vinegar, oil, ginger and black pepper, toss, cover and cook on Low for 6 hours. Divide between plates and serve as a side dish.
Enjoy!

Nutrition: calories 177, fat 2, fiber 7, carbs 11, protein 3

Artichokes Mix

Preparation time: 10 minutes
Cooking time: 5 hours
Servings: 8

Ingredients:
- 4 artichokes, trimmed and halved
- 2 cups whole wheat breadcrumbs
- 1 tablespoon olive oil
- Juice of 1 lemon
- 3 garlic cloves, minced
- 1/3 cup low-fat parmesan, grated
- 1 tablespoon lemon zest, grated
- 2 tablespoons parsley, chopped
- Black pepper to the taste
- 1 cup low-sodium vegetable stock
- 1 tablespoon shallot, minced
- 1 teaspoon oregano, chopped

Directions:
Rub artichokes with the lemon juice and the oil and put them in your slow cooker. Add breadcrumbs, garlic, parsley, parmesan, lemon zest, black pepper, shallot, oregano and stock, cover and cook on Low for 5 hours. Divide the whole mix between plates, sprinkle parsley on top and serve as a side dish.
Enjoy!

Nutrition: calories 200, fat 4, fiber 4, carbs 10, protein 6

Asparagus Mix

Preparation time: 10 minutes
Cooking time: 2 hours
Servings: 4

Ingredients:
- 1 pound asparagus, trimmed and halved
- 1 tablespoon parsley, chopped
- ½ cup low-sodium veggie stock
- 1 garlic clove, minced
- ¼ teaspoon lemon zest, grated
- 2 teaspoons lemon juice

Directions:
In your slow cooker, mix the asparagus with the parsley, stock, garlic, lemon zest and lemon juice, toss a bit, cover and cook on High for 2 hours. Divide the asparagus between plates and serve as a side dish.
Enjoy!

Nutrition: calories 130, fat 3, fiber 2, carbs 10, protein 4

Black Bean and Corn Mix

Preparation time: 10 minutes
Cooking time: 6 hours
Servings: 6

Ingredients:
- 4 tomatoes, chopped
- 1 cup corn kernels
- 16 ounces canned black beans, drained
- 2 garlic cloves, minced
- ½ cup parsley, chopped
- 1 small red onion, chopped
- 1 red bell pepper, chopped
- Juice of 1 lemon
- 2 tablespoons stevia

Directions:
In your slow cooker, mix the tomatoes with corn, black beans, garlic, parsley, lemon juice, bell pepper, onion and stevia, toss, cook on Low for 6 hours, divide between plates and serve as a side dish.
Enjoy!

Nutrition: calories 210, fat 1, fiber 5, carbs 15, protein 7

Celery Mix

Preparation time: 10 minutes
Cooking time: 3 hours
Servings: 3

Ingredients:
- 2 celery roots, cut into medium wedges
- 1 cup low-sodium veggie stock
- 1 teaspoon mustard
- ¼ cup low-fat sour cream
- Black pepper to the taste
- 2 teaspoons thyme, chopped

Directions:
In your slow cooker, mix the celery with the stock, mustard, cream, black pepper and thyme, cover and cook on High for 3 hours. Divide the celery between plates, drizzle some of the cooking juices on top and serve as a side dish.
Enjoy!

Nutrition: calories 160, fat 2, fiber 1, carbs 7, protein 4

Kale Side Dish

Preparation time: 10 minutes
Cooking time: 2 hours
Servings: 6

Ingredients:
- 1 pound kale, chopped
- 2 teaspoons olive oil
- 4 garlic cloves, minced
- ½ cup low-sodium veggie stock
- 1 tablespoons lemon juice
- 1 cup cherry tomatoes, halved
- Black pepper to the taste

Directions:
Heat up a pan with the oil over medium heat, add garlic, stir, cook for 2 minutes and transfer to your slow cooker. Add kale, stock, tomatoes, black pepper and lemon juice, cover, cook on High for 2 hours. Divide the whole mix between plates and serve as a side dish.
Enjoy!

Nutrition: calories 160, fat 2, fiber 3, carbs 8, protein 4

Spicy Eggplant

Preparation time: 10 minutes
Cooking time: 3 hours
Servings: 4

Ingredients:
- 1 eggplant, sliced
- ½ teaspoon cumin, ground
- 1 teaspoon mustard seed
- ½ teaspoon coriander, ground
- ½ teaspoon curry powder
- A pinch of nutmeg, ground
- 2 cups cherry tomatoes, halved
- ½ yellow onion, chopped
- 1 tablespoon olive oil
- 1 garlic clove, minced
- 1 teaspoon red wine vinegar
- Black pepper to the taste
- 1 tablespoon cilantro, chopped

Directions:
Grease the slow cooker with the oil and add eggplant slices inside. Add cumin, mustard seeds, coriander, curry powder, nutmeg, tomatoes, onion, garlic, vinegar, black pepper and cilantro, cover and cook on High for 3 hours. Divide between plates and serve as a side dish.
Enjoy!

Nutrition: calories 180, fat 4, fiber 5, carbs 20, protein 4

Corn Salad

Preparation time: 10 minutes
Cooking time: 2 hours
Servings: 6

Ingredients:
- 2 ounces prosciutto, cut into strips
- 1 teaspoon olive oil
- 2 cups corn
- ½ cup salt-free tomato sauce
- 1 teaspoon garlic, minced
- 1 green bell pepper, chopped

Directions:
Grease your slow cooker with the oil, add corn, prosciutto, tomato sauce, garlic and bell pepper, cover and cook on High for 2 hours. Divide between plates and serve as a side dish.
Enjoy!

Nutrition: calories 109, fat 2, fiber 2, carbs 10, protein 5

Spiced Cabbage

Preparation time: 10 minutes
Cooking time: 4 hours
Servings: 6

Ingredients:
- 2 yellow onions, chopped
- 10 cups red cabbage, shredded
- 1 cup plums, pitted and chopped
- 1 teaspoon cinnamon powder
- 1 garlic clove, minced
- 1 teaspoon cumin seeds
- ¼ teaspoon cloves, ground
- 2 tablespoons red wine vinegar
- 1 teaspoon coriander seeds
- ½ cup water

Directions:
In your slow cooker, mix cabbage with onions, plums, garlic, cinnamon, cumin, cloves, vinegar, coriander and water, stir, cover and cook on Low for 4 hours. Divide between plates and serve as a side dish.
Enjoy!

Nutrition: calories 197, fat 1, fiber 5, carbs 14, protein 3

Spinach and Beans Mix

Preparation time: 10 minutes
Cooking time: 4 hours
Servings: 6

Ingredients:
- 5 carrots, sliced
- 1 and ½ cups great northern beans, dried
- 2 garlic cloves, minced
- 1 yellow onion, chopped
- Black pepper to the taste
- ½ teaspoon oregano, dried
- 5 ounces baby spinach
- 4 and ½ cups low-sodium veggie stock
- 2 teaspoons lemon peel, grated
- 3 tablespoons lemon juice

Directions:
In your slow cooker, mix beans with onion, carrots, garlic, pepper, oregano and stock, stir, cover and cook on High for 4 hours. Add spinach, lemon juice and lemon peel, stir, leave aside for 5 minutes, divide between plates and serve.
Enjoy!

Nutrition: calories 219, fat 8, fiber 14, carbs 14, protein 8

Sage Sweet Potatoes

Preparation time: 10 minutes
Cooking time: 3 hours
Servings: 10

Ingredients:
- 4 pounds sweet potatoes, sliced
- 3 tablespoons stevia
- ½ cup orange juice
- A pinch of black pepper
- ½ teaspoon thyme, dried
- ½ teaspoon sage, dried
- 2 tablespoons olive oil

Directions:
In a bowl, mix orange juice with salt, pepper, stevia, thyme, sage and oil and whisk well. Add the potatoes to your slow cooker, drizzle the sage and orange mix all over, cover, cook on High for 3 hours, divide between plates and serve as a side dish.
Enjoy!

Nutrition: calories 189, fat 4, fiber 4, carbs 16, protein 4

Garlicky Potato Mash

Preparation time: 10 minutes
Cooking time: 4 hours
Servings: 6

Ingredients:
- 6 garlic cloves, peeled
- 3 pounds gold potatoes, peeled and cubed
- 1 bay leaf
- 1 cup coconut milk
- 28 ounces low-sodium veggie stock
- 3 tablespoons olive oil
- Black pepper to the taste

Directions:
In your slow cooker, mix potatoes with stock, bay leaf, garlic, salt and pepper, cover and cook on High for 4 hours. Drain potatoes and garlic, mash them, add oil and milk, whisk well, divide between plates and serve as a side dish.
Enjoy!

Nutrition: calories 135, fat 5, fiber 1, carbs 16, protein 3

Chickpeas Side Dish

Preparation time: 10 minutes
Cooking time: 8 hours
Servings: 6

Ingredients:
- 30 ounces canned chickpeas, no-salt-added, drained and rinsed
- 2 tablespoons olive oil
- 2 tablespoons rosemary, chopped
- A pinch of black pepper
- 2 cups cherry tomatoes, halved
- 2 garlic cloves, minced
- 1 cup corn
- 7 small baby carrots
- 28 ounces low-sodium veggie stock
- 4 cups baby spinach
- 8 ounces zucchini, sliced

Directions:
In your slow cooker, mix chickpeas with oil, rosemary, pepper, cherry tomatoes, garlic, corn, baby carrots, zucchini, spinach and stock, stir, cover, cook on Low for 8 hours, divide between plates and serve.
Enjoy!

Nutrition: calories 203, fat 7, fiber 11, carbs 28, protein 12

Warm Eggplant Salad

Preparation time: 10 minutes
Cooking time: 2 hours
Servings: 6

Ingredients:
- 14 ounces canned roasted tomatoes, no-salt-added and chopped
- 4 cups eggplant, cubed
- 1 yellow bell pepper, chopped
- 1 red onion, cut into medium wedges
- 4 cups kale, torn
- 2 tablespoons olive oil
- 1 teaspoon mustard
- 3 tablespoons red vinegar
- 1 garlic clove, minced
- A pinch of black pepper
- ½ cup parsley, chopped

Directions:
In your slow cooker, mix eggplant with tomatoes, bell pepper and onion, cover and cook on High for 2 hours. In a bowl, mix oil with vinegar, mustard, garlic and pepper, whisk well, add to your slow cooker, also add kale and parsley, toss, divide between plates and serve as a side dish.
Enjoy!

Nutrition: calories 201, fat 9, fiber 6, carbs 16, protein 8

Garlic and Rosemary Potato Mix

Preparation time: 10 minutes
Cooking time: 3 hours
Servings: 12

Ingredients:
- 2 tablespoons olive oil
- 3 pounds baby potatoes, halved
- 7 garlic cloves, minced
- 1 tablespoon rosemary, chopped
- A pinch of black pepper

Directions:
In your slow cooker, mix oil with potatoes, garlic, rosemary and pepper, toss, cover, cook on High for 3 hours, divide between plates and serve.
Enjoy!

Nutrition: calories 192, fat 2, fiber 2, carbs 18, protein 2

Apple Brussels Sprouts

Preparation time: 10 minutes
Cooking time: 3 hours
Servings: 12

Ingredients:
- 1 cup red onion, chopped
- 2 pounds Brussels sprouts, trimmed and halved
- A pinch of black pepper
- ¼ cup natural apple juice, unsweetened
- 3 tablespoons olive oil
- 1 tablespoon cilantro, chopped

Directions:
In your slow cooker, mix Brussels sprouts with onion, oil, cilantro, pepper and apple juice, toss, cover and cook on Low for 3 hours. Toss well, divide between plates and serve as a side dish.
Enjoy!

Nutrition: calories 150, fat 4, fiber 4, carbs 14, protein 3

Italian Beans Mix

Preparation time: 10 minutes
Cooking time: 6 hours
Servings: 8

Ingredients:
- 38 ounces canned cannellini beans, no-salt-added, drained and rinsed
- 1 yellow onion, chopped
- 1 tablespoon olive oil
- ¼ cup basil, chopped
- 19 ounces canned fava beans, no-salt-added, drained and rinsed
- 4 garlic cloves, minced
- 1 and ½ teaspoon Italian seasoning
- 3 tomatoes, chopped
- 2 cups spinach
- 1 cup radicchio, torn

Directions:
In your slow cooker, mix cannellini beans with fava beans, oil, basil, onion, garlic, Italian seasoning, tomato, spinach and radicchio, toss, cover, cook on Low for 6 hours, divide between plates and serve as a side dish.
Enjoy!

Nutrition: calories 264, fat 12, fiber 10, carbs 15, protein 16

Tomatoes, Okra and Zucchini Mix

Preparation time: 10 minutes
Cooking time: 3 hours
Servings: 4

Ingredients:
- 1 and ½ cups red onion, cut into wedges
- 1 cup cherry tomatoes, halved
- 2 cups okra, sliced
- 2 and ½ cups zucchini, sliced
- 2 cups yellow bell pepper, chopped
- 1 cup mushrooms, sliced
- 2 tablespoons basil, chopped
- 1 tablespoon thyme, chopped
- ½ cup olive oil
- ½ cup balsamic vinegar

Directions:
In a large bowl, mix onion with tomatoes, okra, zucchini, bell pepper, mushrooms, basil, thyme, oil and vinegar, cover and cook on High for 3 hours. Divide between plates and serve as a side dish.
Enjoy!

Nutrition: calories 210, fat 2, fiber 2, carbs 6, protein 5

Easy Cabbage

Preparation time: 10 minutes
Cooking time: 6 hours
Servings: 4

Ingredients:
- 1 onion, sliced
- 1 cabbage, shredded
- 2 apples, peeled, cored and roughly chopped
- Black pepper to the taste
- 1 cup low-sodium chicken stock
- 3 tablespoons mustard
- 1 tablespoon olive oil

Directions:
Grease your slow cooker with the oil and add apples, cabbage and onions. In a bowl, mix stock with mustard and black pepper, whisk well, pour this into your slow cooker, cover, cook on Low for 6 hours, divide between plates and serve as a side dish.
Enjoy!

Nutrition: calories 180, fat 4, fiber 2, carbs 5, protein 6

Acorn Squash Mix

Preparation time: 10 minutes
Cooking time: 7 hours
Servings: 4

Ingredients:
- 2 acorn squash, peeled and cut into medium wedges
- 16 ounces canned cranberry sauce, unsweetened
- ¼ teaspoon cinnamon powder
- Black pepper to the taste

Directions:
Put the acorn wedges in your slow cooker; add cranberry sauce, raisins, cinnamon and pepper, stir, cover, cook on Low for 7 hours, divide between plates and serve.
Enjoy!

Nutrition: calories 200, fat 3, fiber 3, carbs 15, protein 2

Italian Zucchini and Squash

Preparation time: 10 minutes
Cooking time: 6 hours
Servings: 6

Ingredients:
- 2 cups zucchinis, sliced
- 1 teaspoon Italian seasoning
- Black pepper to the taste
- 2 cups yellow squash, peeled and cut into wedges
- 1 teaspoon garlic powder
- 2 tablespoons olive oil

Directions:
Grease the slow cooker with the oil, add zucchini, squash, Italian seasoning, black pepper and garlic powder, toss well, cover, cook on Low for 6 hours, divide between plates and serve as a side dish.
Enjoy!

Nutrition: calories 210, fat 2, fiber 4, carbs 16, protein 5

Coconut Broccoli

Preparation time: 10 minutes
Cooking time: 3 hours
Servings: 10

Ingredients:
- 6 cups broccoli florets, chopped
- 10 ounces coconut cream
- ¼ cup yellow onion, chopped
- 1 and ½ cups low-fat cheese, shredded
- 2 tablespoons olive oil

Directions:
Add the oil to your slow cooker, add broccoli, onion, coconut cream, sprinkle cheese, cover and cook on High for 3 hours. Divide between plates and serve as a side dish.
Enjoy!

Nutrition: calories 208, fat 11, fiber 3, carbs 15, protein 5

Asian Green Beans

Preparation time: 10 minutes
Cooking time: 2 hours
Servings: 10

Ingredients:
- 16 cups green beans, halved
- 3 tablespoons olive oil
- ¼ cup tomato sauce, no-salt-added
- ½ cup coconut sugar
- ¾ teaspoon low sodium soy sauce
- A pinch of black pepper

Directions:
In your slow cooker, mix green beans with coconut sugar, tomato sauce, pepper, soy sauce and oil, cover and cook on Low for 3 hours. Divide between plates and serve as a side dish.
Enjoy!

Nutrition: calories 200, fat 4, fiber 5, carbs 12, protein 3

Cauliflower Rice and Mushrooms

Preparation time: 10 minutes
Cooking time: 3 hours
Servings: 6

Ingredients:
- 1 cup cauliflower, riced
- 6 green onions, chopped
- 3 tablespoons olive oil
- 2 garlic cloves, minced
- ½ pound Portobello mushrooms, sliced
- 2 cups water
- A pinch of black pepper

Directions:
In your slow cooker, mix cauliflower with green onions, oil, garlic, mushrooms, water and pepper, stir well, cover, cook on Low for 3 hours, divide between plates and serve as a side dish.
Enjoy!

Nutrition: calories 170, fat 5, fiber 3, carbs 14, protein 4

Cranberries, Cauliflower and Mushroom Mix

Preparation time: 10 minutes
Cooking time: 2 hours and 30 minutes
Servings: 12

Ingredients:
- 1 tablespoons olive oil
- 1 pound mushrooms, sliced
- 6 celery ribs, chopped
- 2 yellow onions, chopped
- 2 garlic cloves, minced
- 1 tablespoon sage, chopped
- 1 cup cranberries, dried
- 1 cup cauliflower florets, chopped
- 1 cup low-sodium veggie stock

Directions:
Add the oil to your slow cooker, add mushrooms, celery, onion, garlic, sage, cranberries, cauliflower and stock, stir, cover and cook on High for 2 hours and 30 minutes. Divide between plates and serve as a side dish.
Enjoy!

Nutrition: calories 193, fat 3, fiber 6, carbs 14, protein 4

Creamy Cauliflower Rice

Preparation time: 10 minutes
Cooking time: 3 hours
Servings: 8

Ingredients:
- 2 garlic cloves, minced
- 2 tablespoons olive oil
- 1 yellow onion, chopped
- ¼ teaspoon thyme, dried
- 3 cups low-sodium veggie stock
- 20 ounces spinach, chopped
- 6 ounces coconut cream
- A pinch of black pepper
- 2 cups cauliflower rice

Directions:
Heat up a pan with the oil over medium heat, add onion, garlic, thyme and stock, stir, cook for 5 minutes and transfer to your slow cooker. Add spinach, coconut cream, cauliflower rice and pepper, cover, cook on High for 3 hours, divide between plates and serve as a side dish.
Enjoy!

Nutrition: calories 187, fat 4, fiber 4, carbs 13, protein 2

Creamy and Cheesy Spinach

Preparation time: 10 minutes
Cooking time: 5 hours
Servings: 6

Ingredients:
- 20 ounces spinach
- 2 cups coconut cream
- 1 cup low-fat cheese, shredded
- 2 tablespoons olive oil

Directions:
In your slow cooker, mix spinach with coconut cream, oil and cheese, cover and cook on Low for 5 hours. Divide between plates and serve as a side dish.
Enjoy!

Nutrition: calories 230, fat 12, fiber 2, carbs 15, protein 12

Dill Cauliflower Mash

Preparation time: 10 minutes
Cooking time: 5 hours
Servings: 6

Ingredients:
- 1 cauliflower head, florets separated
- 1/3 cup dill, chopped
- 6 garlic cloves
- 2 tablespoons olive oil
- A pinch of black pepper

Directions:
Put cauliflower in your slow cooker, add dill, garlic and water to cover them, cover, cook on High for 5 hours, drain, add pepper and oil, mash using a potato masher, whisk well and serve as a side dish.
Enjoy!

Nutrition: calories 207, fat 4, fiber 5, carbs 14, protein 3

Baby Spinach and Avocado Mix

Preparation time: 10 minutes
Cooking time: 4 hours
Servings: 6

Ingredients:
- 5 carrots, sliced
- 2 garlic cloves, minced
- 1 yellow onion, chopped
- A pinch of black pepper
- ½ teaspoon oregano, dried
- 5 ounces baby spinach
- 2 and ½ cups low-sodium veggie stock
- 2 teaspoons lemon peel, grated
- 3 tablespoons lemon juice
- 1 avocado, pitted, peeled and chopped

Directions:
In your slow cooker, mix onion, carrots, garlic, pepper, oregano and stock, stir, cover and cook on High for 4 hours. Add spinach, lemon juice and lemon peel, stir, leave aside for 5 minutes, divide between plates, sprinkle avocado on top and serve as a side dish.
Enjoy!

Nutrition: calories 209, fat 8, fiber 4, carbs 15, protein 17

Simple Parsnips Mix

Preparation time: 10 minutes
Cooking time: 4 hours
Servings: 10

Ingredients:
- 3 pounds parsnips, cut into medium chunks
- 2 tablespoons lemon peel, grated
- 1 cup low-sodium veggie stock
- A pinch of black pepper
- 3 tablespoons olive oil
- ¼ cup cilantro, chopped

Directions:
In your slow cooker, mix parsnips with lemon peel, stock, pepper, oil and cilantro, cover, cook on High for 4 hours, divide between plates and serve as a side dish.
Enjoy!

Nutrition: calories 179, fat 4, fiber 4, carbs 10, protein 5

Basil and Oregano Mushrooms

Preparation time: 10 minutes
Cooking time: 4 hours
Servings: 4

Ingredients:
- 4 garlic cloves, minced
- 24 ounces white mushrooms, halved
- ¼ teaspoon thyme dried
- 1 teaspoon basil, dried
- 1 teaspoon oregano, dried
- 1 cup low-sodium veggie stock
- A pinch of black pepper
- 2 tablespoons olive oil
- 2 tablespoons parsley, chopped

Directions:
Grease the slow cooker with the oil, add mushrooms, garlic, bay leaves, thyme, basil, oregano, black pepper, parsley and stock, cover, cook on Low for 4 hours, divide between plates and serve as a side dish.
Enjoy!

Nutrition: calories 202, fat 6, fiber 1, carbs 14, protein 5

Minty Okra

Preparation time: 10 minutes
Cooking time: 3 hours
Servings: 4

Ingredients:
- 1 pound okra, sliced
- Black pepper to the taste
- 2 tablespoons mint, chopped
- 2 teaspoons olive oil
- 2 tablespoons low-sodium chicken stock
- 4 green onions, chopped

Directions:
Grease your slow cooker with the oil, add okra, pepper, mint, stock and green onions, toss, cover, cook on Low for 3 hours, divide between plates and serve as a side dish.
Enjoy!

Nutrition: calories 130, fat 1, fiber 1, carbs 7, protein 6

Cabbage, Radish and Carrot Mix

Preparation time: 10 minutes
Cooking time: 2 hours
Servings: 6

Ingredients:
- 1 pound green cabbage, chopped
- A pinch of black pepper
- 3 carrots, julienned
- ¼ cup low sodium veggie stock
- 1 cup radish, sliced
- 3 green onion stalks, chopped
- 3 tablespoons chili flakes
- 1 tablespoon olive oil
- ½ inch ginger, grated

Directions:
In your slow cooker, mix cabbage with pepper, carrots, stock, radish, green onions, chili flakes, oil and ginger, toss, cover, cook on High for 2 hours, divide between plates and serve as a side dish.
Enjoy!

Nutrition: calories 170, fat 3, fiber 4, carbs 10, protein 5

Simple Swiss Chard Mix

Preparation time: 10 minutes
Cooking time: 2 hours
Servings: 4

Ingredients:
- 2 tablespoons olive oil
- 3 tablespoons lemon juice
- ½ cup low-sodium veggie stock
- 2 bunches Swiss chard, roughly torn
- ½ teaspoon garlic paste
- Black pepper to the taste

Directions:
In your slow cooker, mix oil with chard, stock, lemon juice, garlic paste and pepper, toss, cover, cook on High for 2 hours, divide between plates and serve.
Enjoy

Nutrition: calories 190, fat 5, fiber 3, carbs 12, protein 4

Dash Diet Slow Cooker Snack and Appetizer Recipes

Eggplant Salsa

Preparation time: 10 minutes
Cooking time: 7 hours
Servings: 4

Ingredients:
- 1 and ½ cups tomatoes, chopped
- 3 cups eggplant, cubed
- 6 ounces green olives, pitted and sliced
- 4 garlic cloves, minced
- 2 teaspoons balsamic vinegar
- 1 tablespoon oregano, chopped
- Black pepper to the taste

Directions:
In your slow cooker, mix tomatoes with eggplant, green olives, garlic, vinegar, oregano and pepper, toss, cover, cook on Low for 7 hours, divide into small bowls and serve as an appetizer. Enjoy!

Nutrition: calories 190, fat 6, fiber 5, carbs 12, protein 2

Artichoke and Beans Spread

Preparation time: 10 minutes
Cooking time: 30 minutes
Servings: 8

Ingredients:
- 4 cups spinach, chopped
- 2 cups artichoke hearts
- Black pepper to the taste
- 1 teaspoon thyme, chopped
- 2 garlic cloves, minced
- 1 cup white beans, already cooked
- 1 tablespoon parsley, chopped
- 2 tablespoons low-fat parmesan, grated
- ½ cup low-fat sour cream

Directions:
In your slow cooker, mix artichokes with spinach, black pepper, thyme, garlic, beans, parmesan, parsley and sour cream, stir, cover and cook on Low for 5 hours. Transfer to your blender, pulse well divide into bowls and serve.
Enjoy!

Nutrition: calories 180, fat 2, fiber 6, carbs 11, protein 5

Stuffed White Mushrooms

Preparation time: 10 minutes
Cooking time: 5 hours
Servings: 20

Ingredients:
- 20 mushrooms, stems removed
- ¼ cup low-fat butter, melted
- 1 and ½ cups whole wheat breadcrumbs
- 2 tablespoons parsley, chopped
- 2 cups basil, chopped
- 1 cup tomato sauce, no-salt-added
- ¼ cup low-fat parmesan, grated
- 1 tablespoon garlic, minced
- 2 teaspoons lemon juice
- 1 tablespoon olive oil

Directions:
In a bowl, mix butter with breadcrumbs and parsley, stir well and leave aside. In your blender, mix basil with oil, parmesan, garlic and lemon juice and pulse really well. Stuff mushrooms with this mix, pour the tomato sauce on top, sprinkle breadcrumbs mix at the end, cover and cook on Low for 5 hours. Arrange mushrooms on a platter and serve.
Enjoy!

Nutrition: calories 170, fat 1, fiber 3, carbs 14, protein 4

Italian Tomato Appetizer

Preparation time: 10 minutes
Cooking time: 2 hours
Servings: 4

Ingredients:
- 2 teaspoons olive oil
- 8 tomatoes, chopped
- ¼ cup basil, chopped
- 3 tablespoons low-sodium veggie stock
- 1 garlic clove, minced
- 4 Italian whole wheat bread slices, toasted
- Black pepper to the taste

Directions:
In your slow cooker, mix tomatoes with basil, garlic, oil, stock and black pepper, stir, cover, cook on High for 2 hours and then leave aside to cool down. Divide this mix on the toasted bread and serve as an appetizer.
Enjoy!

Nutrition: calories 174, fat 2, fiber 1, carbs 10, protein 4

Sweet Pineapple Snack

Preparation time: 10 minutes
Cooking time: 2 hours
Servings: 8

Ingredients:
- 1 tablespoon lime juice
- 2 tablespoons honey
- 1 tablespoon olive oil
- 1 teaspoon cinnamon powder
- 1 pineapple, peeled and cut into medium sticks
- ¼ teaspoon cloves, ground
- 1 tablespoon lime zest, grated

Directions:
In a bowl, mix lime juice with honey, oil, cinnamon and cloves and whisk well. Add the pineapple sticks to your slow cooker, add lime mix, toss, cover and cook on High for 2 hours. Serve the pineapple sticks as a snack with lime zest sprinkled on top.
Enjoy!

Nutrition: calories 130, fat 4, fiber 1, carbs 10, protein 3

Chickpeas Hummus

Preparation time: 10 minutes
Cooking time: 5 hours
Servings: 6

Ingredients:
- 1 cup chickpeas, soaked overnight and drained
- 2 garlic cloves
- 3 cups water
- 1 tablespoon olive oil
- 2 tablespoons sherry vinegar
- ¾ cup green onions, chopped
- 1 teaspoon cumin, ground
- 3 tablespoons cilantro, chopped

Directions:
Put the water in your slow cooker, add chickpeas and garlic, cover and cook on Low for 5 hours. Drain chickpeas, transfer them to your blender, add ½ cup of the cooking liquid, green onions, vinegar, oil, cilantro and cumin, blend well, divide into bowls and serve.
Enjoy!

Nutrition: calories 133, fat 1, fiber 3, carbs 10, protein 3

Asparagus Snack

Preparation time: 4 weeks
Cooking time: 2 hours
Servings: 6

Ingredients:
- 3 cups asparagus spears, halved
- ¼ cup apple cider vinegar
- 1 tablespoon dill
- ¼ cup white wine vinegar
- 2 cloves
- 1 cup water
- 3 garlic cloves, sliced
- ¼ teaspoon red pepper flakes
- 8 black peppercorns
- 1 teaspoon coriander seeds

Directions:
In your slow cooker, mix the asparagus with the cider vinegar, white vinegar, dill, cloves, water, garlic, pepper flakes, peppercorns and coriander, cover and cook on High for 2 hours. Drain asparagus, transfer it to bowls and serve as a snack.
Enjoy!

Nutrition: calories 90, fat 1, fiber 2, carbs 7, protein 2

Shrimp and Beans Appetizer Salad

Preparation time: 10 minutes
Cooking time: 5 hours and 30 minutes.
Servings: 8

Ingredients:
- ¼ pound shrimp, peeled, deveined and chopped
- Zest and juice of 2 limes
- Zest and juice of 2 lemons
- 2 teaspoons cumin, ground
- 2 tablespoons olive oil
- 1 cup tomato, chopped
- ½ cup red onion, chopped
- 2 tablespoons garlic, minced
- 1 cup canned black beans, no-salt-added, drained and rinsed
- 1 cup cucumber, chopped
- ¼ cup cilantro, chopped

Directions:
In a bowl, mix limejuice and lemon juice with shrimp and toss. Grease the slow cooker with the oil, add black beans, tomato, onion, garlic and cumin, cover and cook on Low for 5 hours. Add shrimp, cover, cook on Low for 30 minutes, more, transfer everything to a bowl, add cucumber and cilantro, toss, leave aside to cool down, divide between small bowls and serve as an appetizer.
Enjoy!

Nutrition: calories 200, fat 3, fiber 2, carbs 15, protein 5

Pepper and Chickpeas Dip

Preparation time: 10 minutes
Cooking time: 2 hours
Servings: 12

Ingredients:
- 1 cup red bell pepper, sliced
- 1 tablespoon olive oil
- 2 tablespoons white sesame seeds
- 2 cups canned chickpeas, no-salt-added, drained and rinsed
- 1 tablespoon lemon juice
- 1 teaspoon garlic powder
- 1 teaspoon onion powder
- A pinch of cayenne pepper
- 1 and ¼ teaspoons cumin, ground

Directions:
In your slow cooker, mix red bell pepper with oil, sesame seeds, chickpeas, lemon juice, garlic and onion powder, cayenne pepper and cumin, cover and cook on High for 2 hours. Transfer this mix to your blender, pulse well, divide into serving bowls and serve cold.
Enjoy!

Nutrition: calories 180, fat 2, fiber 2, carbs 15, protein 3

White Bean Spread

Preparation time: 10 minutes
Cooking time: 6 hours
Servings: 8

Ingredients:
- 15 ounces canned white beans, no-salt-added, drained and rinsed
- 1 cup low-sodium veggie stock
- 2 tablespoons olive oil
- 8 garlic cloves, roasted
- 2 tablespoons lemon juice

Directions:
In your blender, mix beans with oil, stock, garlic and lemon juice, cover, cook on Low for 6 hours, transfer to your blender, pulse well, divide into bowls and serve as a snack.
Enjoy!

Nutrition: calories 159, fat 4, fiber 3, carbs 14, protein 2

Minty Spinach Dip

Preparation time: 20 minutes
Cooking time: 2 hours
Servings: 4

Ingredients:
- 1 bunch spinach leaves, roughly chopped
- 1 scallion, sliced
- 2 tablespoons mint leaves, chopped
- ¾ cup low-fat sour cream
- Black pepper to the taste

Directions:
In your slow cooker, mix the spinach with the scallion, mint, cream and black pepper, cover, and cook on High for 2 hours, stir well, divide into bowls and serve.
Enjoy!

Nutrition: calories 160, fat 3, fiber 3, carbs 12, protein 5

Turnips and Cauliflower Spread

Preparation time: 10 minutes
Cooking time: 7 hours
Servings: 4

Ingredients:
- 2 cups cauliflower florets
- 1/3 cup cashews, chopped
- 1 cup turnips, chopped
- 2 and ½ cups water
- 1 cup coconut milk
- 1 teaspoon garlic powder
- ¼ teaspoon smoked paprika
- ¼ teaspoon mustard powder

Directions:
In your slow cooker, mix cauliflower with cashews, turnips and water, stir, cover, cook on Low for 7 hours, drain, transfer to a blender, add milk, garlic powder, paprika and mustard powder, blend well, divide into bowls and serve as a snack
Enjoy!

Nutrition: calories 221, fat 7, fiber 4, carbs 14, protein 3

Italian Veggie Dip

Preparation time: 10 minutes
Cooking time: 5 hours
Servings: 7

Ingredients:
- ½ cauliflower head, riced
- 54 ounces canned tomatoes, no-salt-added and crushed
- 10 ounces white mushrooms, chopped
- 3 cups eggplant, cubed
- 6 garlic cloves, minced
- 2 tablespoons stevia
- 2 tablespoons balsamic vinegar
- 2 tablespoons tomato paste, no-salt-added
- 1 tablespoon basil, chopped
- 1 and ½ tablespoons oregano, chopped
- A pinch of black pepper

Directions:
In your slow cooker, mix cauliflower with tomatoes, mushrooms, eggplant, garlic, stevia, vinegar, tomato paste and pepper, stir, cover and cook on High for 5 hours. Add basil and oregano, stir, mash a bit with a potato masher, divide into bowls and serve as a dip.
Enjoy!

Nutrition: calories 261, fat 7, fiber 6, carbs 11, protein 6

Cajun Peas Spread

Preparation time: 10 minutes
Cooking time: 5 hours
Servings: 5

Ingredients:
- 1 and ½ cups black-eyed peas
- 3 cups water
- 1 teaspoon Cajun seasoning
- ½ cup pecans, toasted
- ½ teaspoon garlic powder
- ½ teaspoon chili powder
- A pinch of black pepper
- ½ teaspoon Tabasco sauce

Directions:
In your slow cooker, mix the peas with Cajun seasoning, pepper and water, stir, cover and cook on High for 5 hours. Drain, transfer to a blender, add pecans, garlic powder, chili powder and Tabasco sauce, pulse well, divide into bowls and serve as a snack
Enjoy!

Nutrition: calories 241, fat 4, fiber 7, carbs 12, protein 4

Cashew Spread

Preparation time: 10 minutes
Cooking time: 3 hours
Servings: 10

Ingredients:
- 1 cup water
- 1 cup cashews
- 10 ounces hummus, no-salt-added
- ¼ teaspoon garlic powder
- ¼ teaspoon onion powder
- A pinch of black pepper
- 1 teaspoon apple cider vinegar

Directions:
In your slow cooker, mix water with cashews and pepper, stir, cover, cook on High for 3 hours, transfer to your blender, add hummus, garlic powder, onion powder and vinegar, pulse well, divide into bowls and serve.
Enjoy!

Nutrition: calories 212, fat 7, fiber 7, carbs 15, protein 4

Coconut Spinach Dip

Preparation time: 10 minutes
Cooking time: 1 hour
Servings: 4

Ingredients:
- 1 cup coconut cream
- 10 ounces spinach leaves
- 8 ounces water chestnuts, chopped
- 1 garlic clove, minced
- Black pepper to the taste

Directions:
In your slow cooker, mix coconut cream with spinach, chestnuts, black pepper and garlic, stir, cover, cook on High for 1 hour, blend with an immersion blender, divide into bowls and serve as a dip
Enjoy!

Nutrition: calories 192, fat 5, fiber 7, carbs 12, protein 5

Black Bean Salsa

Preparation time: 10 minutes
Cooking time: 4 hours
Servings: 7

Ingredients:
- 1 tablespoon low sodium soy sauce
- ½ teaspoon cumin, ground
- 1 cup canned black beans, no-salt-added, drained and rinsed
- 1 cup chunky salsa, salt-free
- 6 cups romaine lettuce, torn
- ½ cup avocado, peeled, pitted and mashed

Directions:
In your slow cooker, mix the beans with salsa, cumin and soy sauce, stir, cover and cook on Low for 4 hours. In a salad bowl, mix lettuce leaves with black beans mix and mashed avocado, toss, divide into small bowls and serve.
Enjoy!

Nutrition: calories 199, fat 4, fiber 7, carbs 14, protein 4

Chili Coconut Corn Spread

Preparation time: 10 minutes
Cooking time: 2 hours
Servings: 8

Ingredients:
- 30 ounces canned corn, no-salt-added, drained
- 2 green onions, chopped
- ½ cup coconut cream
- 8 ounces low-fat cream cheese
- 1 jalapeno, chopped
- ½ teaspoon chili powder

Directions:
In your slow cooker, mix corn with green onions, coconut cream, cream cheese, chili powder and jalapeno, cover, cook on Low for 2 hours, whisk well, divide into bowls and serve as a dip.
Enjoy!

Nutrition: calories 302, fat 5, fiber 7, carbs 12, protein 4

Artichoke and Spinach Dip

Preparation time: 10 minutes
Cooking time: 2 hours
Servings: 8

Ingredients:
- 28 ounces canned artichokes, no-salt-added, drained and chopped
- 10 ounces spinach
- 8 ounces coconut cream
- 1 yellow onion, chopped
- 2 garlic cloves, minced
- ¾ cup coconut milk
- 3 tablespoons avocado mayonnaise
- 1 tablespoon red vinegar
- A pinch of black pepper

Directions:
In your slow cooker, mix artichokes with spinach, cream, onion, garlic, milk, mayo, vinegar and pepper, stir, cover, cook on Low for 2 hours, divide into bowls and serve as a snack.
Enjoy!

Nutrition: calories 255, fat 7, fiber 4, carbs 20, protein 13

Mushroom and Bell Pepper Dip

Preparation time: 10 minutes
Cooking time: 4 hours
Servings: 6

Ingredients:
- 3 cups green bell peppers, chopped
- 1 red onion, chopped
- 3 garlic cloves, minced
- 1 pound mushrooms, chopped
- 28 ounces tomato sauce, no-salt-added
- ½ cup low-fat cheddar, grated
- Black pepper to the taste

Directions:
In your slow cooker, mix bell peppers with mushrooms, onion, garlic, tomato sauce, cheese and pepper, stir, cover, cook on Low for 4 hours, divide into bowls and serve.
Enjoy!

Nutrition: calories 253, fat 4, fiber 7, carbs 15, protein 3

Warm French Veggie Salad

Preparation time: 10 minutes
Cooking time: 9 hours
Servings: 6

Ingredients:
- 2 yellow onions, chopped
- 1 eggplant, sliced
- 4 zucchinis, sliced
- 2 garlic cloves, minced
- 2 green bell peppers, cut into medium strips
- 6 ounces canned tomato paste, no-salt-added
- 2 tomatoes, cut into medium wedges
- 1 teaspoon oregano, dried
- 1 tablespoon basil, chopped
- 2 tablespoons parsley, chopped
- 3 tablespoons olive oil
- A pinch of black pepper

Directions:
In your slow cooker, mix oil with onions, eggplant, zucchinis, garlic, bell peppers, tomato paste, tomatoes, basil, oregano and pepper, cover and cook on Low for 9 hours. Add parsley, toss, divide into small bowls and serve warm as an appetizer.
Enjoy!

Nutrition: calories 219, fat 7, fiber 6, carbs 18, protein 4

Bulgur and Beans Salad

Preparation time: 10 minutes
Cooking time: 8 hours
Servings: 4

Ingredients:
- 2 cups white mushrooms, sliced
- ¾ cup bulgur, soaked and drained
- 2 cups yellow onion, chopped
- ½ cup red bell pepper, chopped
- 1 cup low sodium veggie stock
- 2 garlic cloves, minced
- 1 cup strong coffee
- 14 ounces canned kidney beans, no-salt-added, drained
- 14 ounces canned pinto beans, no-salt-added, drained
- 2 tablespoons stevia
- 2 tablespoons chili powder
- 1 tablespoon cocoa powder
- 1 teaspoon oregano, dried
- 2 teaspoons cumin, ground
- Black pepper to the taste

Directions:
In your slow cooker, mix mushrooms with bulgur, onion, bell pepper, stock, garlic, coffee, kidney and pinto beans, stevia, chili powder, cocoa, oregano, cumin and pepper, stir gently, cover and cook on Low for 12 hours. Divide the mix into small bowls and serve cold as an appetizer.
Enjoy!

Nutrition: calories 301, fat 4, fiber 6, carbs 16, protein 4

Pineapple Chicken Wings

Preparation time: 10 minutes
Cooking time: 3 hours
Servings: 6

Ingredients:
- 2 tablespoons garlic, minced
- 2 and ¼ cups pineapple juice, unsweetened
- 3 tablespoons low sodium soy sauce
- 2 tablespoons almond flour
- 1 tablespoon ginger, minced
- 1 teaspoon olive oil
- 3 pounds chicken wings
- A pinch of red pepper flakes, crushed
- 2 tablespoons 5 spice powder

Directions:
Put the pineapple juice in your slow cooker, add the oil, ginger, soy sauce, garlic and flour and whisk really well. Season chicken wings with pepper flakes and 5-spice powder, add them to your slow cooker, cover and cook on High for 3 hours. Transfer chicken wings to a platter, drizzle some of the sauce over them and serve as an appetizer.
Enjoy!

Nutrition: calories 199, fat 4, fiber 4, carbs 13, protein 16

Spiced Pecans Snack

Preparation time: 10 minutes
Cooking time: 2 hours
Servings: 5

Ingredients:
- 1 pound pecans, halved
- 2 tablespoons olive oil
- 1 teaspoon basil, dried
- 1 tablespoon chili powder
- 1 teaspoon oregano, dried
- ¼ teaspoon garlic powder
- 1 teaspoon rosemary, dried
- ½ teaspoon onion powder

Directions:
In your slow cooker, mix pecans with oil, basil, chili powder, oregano, garlic powder, onion powder and rosemary, toss, cover and cook on Low for 2 hours. Divide into bowls and serve as a snack.
Enjoy!

Nutrition: calories 152, fat 3, fiber 2, carbs 11, protein 2

Easy Pork Party Meatballs

Preparation time: 10 minutes
Cooking time: 4 hours
Servings: 4

Ingredients:
- 1 and ½ pounds pork, minced
- 2 small yellow onions, chopped
- 1 egg, whisked
- Black pepper to the taste
- 3 tablespoons cilantro, chopped
- 14 ounces coconut milk
- 2 tablespoons hot sauce
- 1 teaspoon basil, dried
- 1 tablespoon green curry paste
- 1 tablespoon low sodium soy sauce

Directions:
Put the meat in a bowl, add onion, egg, pepper and cilantro, stir well, shape medium-sized meatballs and place them in your slow cooker. Add hot sauce, soy sauce, milk, curry paste and basil, toss and cook on Low for 4 hours. Arrange meatballs on a platter and serve them as an appetizer.
Enjoy!

Nutrition: calories 200, fat 6, fiber 2, carbs 14, protein 4

Pork Rolls

Preparation time: 10 minutes
Cooking time: 8 hours
Servings: 4

Ingredients:
- ½ pounds pork meat, minced
- 1 green cabbage head, leaves separated
- ½ cup onion, chopped
- 1 cup cauliflower rice
- 2 ounces white mushrooms, chopped
- 2 garlic cloves, minced
- 2 tablespoons dill, chopped
- 1 tablespoon olive oil
- 25 ounces tomato sauce, no-salt-added
- A pinch of black pepper
- ¼ cup water

Directions:
In a bowl, mix pork with onion, cauliflower, mushrooms, garlic, dill and pepper and stir. Arrange cabbage leaves on a working surface, divide the pork mix and wrap them well. Add sauce and water to your slow cooker, stir, add cabbage rolls, cover, cook on Low for 8 hours, arrange the rolls on a platter and serve them as an appetizer.
Enjoy!

Nutrition: calories 301, fat 6, fiber 6, carbs 16, protein 8

Tomato Salsa

Preparation time: 10 minutes
Cooking time: 7 hours
Servings: 4

Ingredients:
- 3 cups tomatoes, chopped
- 2 teaspoons capers, no-salt-added
- 8 ounces black olives, pitted and sliced
- 1 red onion, chopped
- 2 teaspoons balsamic vinegar
- 2 tablespoons mint, chopped
- Black pepper to the taste

Directions:
In your slow cooker, mix tomatoes with capers, olives, onion, vinegar, mint and pepper, toss, cover and cook on Low for 7 hours. Divide salsa into small bowls and serve cold.
Enjoy!

Nutrition: calories 200, fat 6, fiber 5, carbs 16, protein 2

White Fish Sticks

Preparation time: 10 minutes
Cooking time: 2 hours
Servings: 4

Ingredients:
- 2 eggs
- 1 pound white fish fillets, skinless, boneless and cut into medium strips
- Black pepper to the taste
- 1 cup almond flour
- ¼ teaspoon paprika
- Cooking spray

Directions:
In a bowl, mix the flour with pepper and paprika and stir. Put the eggs in another bowl and whisk them well. Dip fish sticks in the egg, dredge in flour mix, arrange them in your slow cooker greased with cooking spray, cover and cook on High for 2 hours. Serve them as an appetizer.
Enjoy!

Nutrition: calories 221, fat 2, fiber 4, carbs 15, protein 10

Tomato Shrimp Salad

Preparation time: 10 minutes
Cooking time: 3 hours
Servings: 4

Ingredients:
- 3 pounds shrimp, peeled and deveined
- 1 red onion, chopped
- 14 ounces canned tomato paste, no-salt-added

Directions:
In your slow cooker, mix shrimp with onion and tomato paste, stir, cover and cook on Low for 3 hours. Divide into small bowls and serve.
Enjoy!

Nutrition: calories 211, fat 2, fiber 7, carbs 17, protein 5

Stuffed Chicken

Preparation time: 10 minutes
Cooking time: 6 hours
Servings: 4

Ingredients:
- 4 chicken breasts, skinless and boneless
- 1 tablespoon olive oil
- 1 small yellow onion, chopped
- 2 chili peppers, chopped
- 1 red bell pepper, chopped
- 2 teaspoons garlic, minced
- 6 ounces spinach
- 1 tablespoon lemon juice
- 1 cup low-sodium veggie stock
- A pinch of black pepper
- A handful parsley, chopped

Directions:
Heat up a pan with the oil over medium-high heat, add bell pepper, chili peppers, onions, spinach, garlic, pepper and oregano, stir, cook for a couple of minutes and take off heat. Cut a pocket in each chicken breast, stuff with spinach mix, arrange in your slow cooker, add the stock, cover, cook on Low for 6 hours, arrange stuffed chicken on a platter, sprinkle parsley on top, drizzle the lemon juice and serve as an appetizer.
Enjoy!

Nutrition: calories 225, fat 4, fiber 3, carbs 15, protein 11

Italian Nuts Mix

Preparation time: 10 minutes
Cooking time: 4 hours
Servings: 20

Ingredients:
- 4 tablespoons olive oil
- 1-ounce Italian seasoning
- 1 teaspoon cinnamon powder
- Cayenne pepper to the taste
- 2 cups cashews
- 2 cups almonds
- 2 cups walnuts

Directions:
In your slow cooker, mix oil with Italian seasoning, cinnamon, cayenne, cashews, almonds and walnuts, toss well, cover, cook on Low for 4 hours, divide into bowls and serve as a snack. Enjoy!

Nutrition: calories 190, fat 4, fiber 3, carbs 7, protein 4

Dill Walnuts and Seeds Mix

Preparation time: 10 minutes
Cooking time: 3 hours
Servings: 10

Ingredients:
- Cooking spray
- 1 cup walnuts, chopped
- 1 cup pumpkin seeds
- 2 tablespoons dill, dried
- 2 tablespoons olive oil
- 1 teaspoon rosemary, dried
- 1 tablespoon lemon peel, grated

Directions:
Spray your slow cooker with cooking spray, add walnuts, pumpkin seeds, oil, dill, rosemary and lemon peel, toss, cover, cook on Low for 3 hours, divide into bowls and serve as a snack. Enjoy!

Nutrition: calories 161, fat 2, fiber 2, carbs 13, protein 2

Tomato Dip

Preparation time: 10 minutes
Cooking time: 5 hours
Servings: 12

Ingredients:
- 8 pounds tomatoes, peeled and chopped
- 2 sweet onions, chopped
- 6 ounces tomato paste, no-salt-added
- ¼ cup white vinegar
- 2 tablespoons stevia
- 1 and ½ tablespoons Italian seasoning
- A pinch of black pepper
- ½ cup basil, chopped

Directions:
In your slow cooker, mix the tomatoes with onions, tomato paste, vinegar, stevia, Italian seasoning, pepper and basil, stir, cover, cook on High for 5 hours, blend using an immersion blender, divide into bowls and serve as a dip.
Enjoy!

Nutrition: calories 182, fat 3, fiber 6, carbs 8, protein 3

Zucchini Dip

Preparation time: 10 minutes
Cooking time: 2 hours
Servings: 4

Ingredients:
- 4 cups zucchinis, chopped
- 1 cup low-sodium chicken stock
- ¼ cup olive oil
- Black pepper to the taste
- 4 garlic cloves, minced
- ¾ cup sesame paste
- ½ cup lemon juice

Directions:
In your slow cooker, mix the zucchinis with stock and pepper, cover, cook on High for 2 hours, transfer to your blender, add oil, garlic, lemon juice and sesame paste, blend, divide into small bowls and serve.
Enjoy!

Nutrition: calories 162, fat 5, fiber 3, carbs 15, protein 7

Easy Zucchini Rolls

Preparation time: 10 minutes
Cooking time: 1 hour
Servings: 24

Ingredients:
- 2 tablespoons olive oil
- 3 zucchinis, thinly sliced
- ½ cup tomato sauce, no-salt-added
- 24 basil leaves
- 2 tablespoons mint, chopped
- 1 and ½ cup low-fat ricotta cheese
- Black pepper to the taste
- ¼ cup basil leaves, whole

Directions:
Brush zucchini slices with half of the olive oil, season with the pepper and place them on a working surface. In a bowl, mix ricotta with chopped basil, mint and pepper, stir well, spread this over zucchini, divide whole basil leaves, roll them, transfer to your slow cooker add the rest of the oil and the tomato sauce, cover, cook on High for 1 hour, arrange them on a platter and serve.
Enjoy!

Nutrition: calories 250, fat 3, fiber 3, carbs 15, protein 2

Jumbo Shrimp Appetizer

Preparation time: 10 minutes
Cooking time: 1 hour
Servings: 4

Ingredients:
- 1 pound jumbo shrimp, peeled and deveined
- 4 teaspoons Worcestershire sauce, salt-free
- 4 teaspoons avocado oil
- 1 and ½ cups low-sodium chicken stock
- Juice of 1 lemon
- Black pepper to the taste
- 2 teaspoons Creole seasoning

Directions:
Grease your slow cooker with the oil, add shrimp, Worcestershire sauce, stock, lemon juice, pepper and Creole seasoning, cover, cook on High for 1 hour, transfer the shrimp to a platter and serve as an appetizer.
Enjoy!

Nutrition: calories 190, fat 3, fiber 1, carbs 12, protein 6

Salmon Appetizer Salad

Preparation time: 10 minutes
Cooking time: 1 hour
Servings: 4

Ingredients:

- 4 medium salmon fillets, boneless and cubed
- 1 cup low sodium veggie stock
- Black pepper to the taste
- 2 shallots, chopped
- 1 lettuce head, torn
- 2 tablespoons lemon juice
- ¼ cup olive oil+ 1 tablespoon
- 3 tablespoons parsley, finely chopped

Directions:
Brush salmon fillets with 1 tablespoon of oil, season with pepper, put them in your slow cooker, add stock, cover and cook on High for 1 hour. Transfer salmon to a salad bowl, add shallots, lemon juice, lettuce, the rest of the oil and parsley, toss and serve as an appetizer.
Enjoy!

Nutrition: calories 210, fat 10, fiber 1, carbs 15, protein 8

Beet and Celery Spread

Preparation time: 10 minutes
Cooking time: 4 hours
Servings: 8

Ingredients:

- 1 yellow onion, chopped
- 2 tablespoons olive oil
- 7 celery ribs
- 8 garlic cloves, minced
- 6 beets, peeled and chopped
- 1 cup low-sodium veggie stock
- ¼ cup lemon juice
- 1 bunch basil, chopped
- Black pepper to the taste

Directions:
Grease your slow cooker with the oil, add celery, onion, beets, garlic, stock, lemon juice, basil and pepper, stir, cover and cook on Low for 4 hours. Blend using an immersion blender, divide into bowls and serve.
Enjoy!

Nutrition: calories 203, fat 1, fiber 3, carbs 13, protein 3

Clams Salad

Preparation time: 10 minutes
Cooking time: 2 hours
Servings: 4

Ingredients:
- 40 small clams
- 1 yellow onion, chopped
- 10 ounces low sodium veggie stock
- 2 tablespoons parsley, chopped
- 1 teaspoon olive oil
- Lemon wedges for serving

Directions:
Grease your slow cooker with the oil; add onion, clams, stock and parsley, toss, cover and cook on High for 2 hours. Divide into small bowls and serve with lemon wedges on the side.
Enjoy!

Nutrition: calories 202, fat 4, fiber 3, carbs 14, protein 6

Creamy Endive Salad

Preparation time: 10 minutes
Cooking time: 3 hours
Servings: 4

Ingredients:
- 4 endives, trimmed
- 1 cup low-sodium chicken stock
- Black pepper to the taste
- 2 tablespoons olive oil
- 4 slices low-sodium ham, chopped
- ½ teaspoon nutmeg, ground
- 14 ounces coconut cream

Directions:
In your slow cooker, mix endives with stock, pepper, oil, ham, nutmeg and coconut cream, cover and cook on High for 3 hours. Divide into small bowls and serve as an appetizer.
Enjoy!

Nutrition: calories 202, fat 3, fiber 3, carbs 14, protein 12

Chili Cauliflower Dip

Preparation time: 10 minutes
Cooking time: 2 hours and 15 minutes
Servings: 6

Ingredients:
- 2 jalapenos, chopped
- ½ cup coconut cream
- 2 cups cauliflower rice
- ¼ cup low-fat cheddar cheese, grated
- A pinch of black pepper
- 2 tablespoons chives, chopped

Directions:
In your slow cooker, mix the jalapenos with the coconut cream, cauliflower, pepper, cheese and chives, stir, cover and cook on Low for 2 hours and 15 minutes. Divide into bowls and serve. Enjoy!

Nutrition: calories 202, fat 3, fiber 3, carbs 14, protein 6

Cranberries, Apple and Onion Salad

Preparation time: 10 minutes
Cooking time: 6 hours
Servings: 12

Ingredients:
- 1 apple, peeled, cored and cut into wedges
- 2 cups sweet onions, sliced
- 2 tablespoons olive oil
- ½ cup cranberries
- ¼ cup balsamic vinegar
- 1 tablespoon stevia
- ½ teaspoon orange zest, grated
- 7 ounces low-fat cheddar cheese, shredded

Directions:
In your slow cooker, mix apples with cranberries, onions, oil, vinegar, stevia and orange zest, stir, cover and cook on Low for 6 hours. Divide into bowls, sprinkle the cheese on top and serve. Enjoy!

Nutrition: calories 142, fat 2, fiber 1, carbs 8, protein 4

Sausage Meatballs and Apricot Sauce

Preparation time: 10 minutes
Cooking time: 5 hours
Servings: 20

Ingredients:
- 2 pounds pork sausage, ground
- 2 eggs
- ½ cup yellow onion, chopped
- 2 tablespoons parsley, chopped
- A pinch of black pepper
- ½ teaspoon garlic powder
- 12 ounces canned apricot preserves, unsweetened

Directions:
In a bowl, mix pork sausage meat with eggs, onion, parsley, pepper and garlic powder, stir well and shape small meatballs out of this mix. Put the meatballs in your slow cooker, add apricot preserves, toss, cover and cook on Low for 5 hours. Arrange meatballs, sauce on a platter, and serve them.
Enjoy!

Nutrition: calories 216, fat 4, fiber 4, carbs 13, protein 4

Sriracha Chicken Dip

Preparation time: 10 minutes
Cooking time: 3 hours and 30 minutes
Servings: 10

Ingredients:
- 1 pound chicken breast, skinless, boneless and sliced
- 3 tablespoons sriracha sauce
- ¼ cup low-sodium chicken stock
- 2 tablespoons stevia
- 1 teaspoon hot sauce, no-salt-added
- 8 ounces coconut cream

Directions:
In your slow cooker, mix chicken with sriracha sauce, stock, stevia and hot sauce, stir, cover and cook on High for 3 hours. Shred meat, return to pot, add coconut cream, cover, cook on High for 30 minutes more, divide into bowls and serve.
Enjoy!

Nutrition: calories 271, fat 5, fiber 6, carbs 16, protein 3

Shrimp Cocktail

Preparation time: 10 minutes
Cooking time: 2 hours and 30 minutes
Servings: 4

Ingredients:
- 1 cup low-sodium chicken stock
- 2 tablespoons olive oil
- 2 teaspoons parsley, chopped
- 2 teaspoons garlic, minced
- 40 shrimp, peeled and deveined

Directions:
In your slow cooker, mix stock with oil, parsley, garlic and shrimp, toss, cover and cook on Low for 2 hours and 30 minutes. Divide into bowls and serve as an appetizer.
Enjoy!

Nutrition: calories 162, fat 2, fiber 6, carbs 9, protein 2

Cod Salsa

Preparation time: 10 minutes
Cooking time: 1 hour and 30 minutes
Servings: 4

Ingredients:
- 1 pound cod fillets, skinless, boneless and cubed
- 1 yellow onion, chopped
- 1 red bell pepper, chopped
- 15 ounces canned tomatoes, no-salt-added and chopped
- 1 tablespoons rosemary, chopped
- ¼ cup low sodium veggie stock

Directions:
In your slow cooker, mix tomatoes with onion, bell pepper, rosemary and stock and stir. Add fish, cover and cook on Low for 1 hour and 30 minutes. Divide everything into bowls and serve warm as an appetizer.
Enjoy!

Nutrition: calories 200, fat 4, fiber 3, carbs 15, protein 4

Salmon and Carrots Appetizer Salad

Preparation time: 10 minutes
Cooking time: 9 hours
Servings: 4

Ingredients:
- 16 ounces baby carrots
- 3 tablespoons olive oil
- 4 garlic cloves, minced
- ¼ cup low-sodium veggie stock
- 4 salmon fillets, boneless and cubed
- ½ teaspoon dill, chopped
- A pinch of black pepper

Directions:
In your slow cooker, mix oil with carrots, stock and garlic, stir, cover and cook on Low for 7 hours. Add salmon, pepper and dill, cover, cook on Low for 2 hours more, divide everything into bowls and serve as an appetizer
Enjoy!

Nutrition: calories 212, fat 3, fiber 6, carbs 15, protein 6

Italian Shrimp Salad

Preparation time: 10 minutes
Cooking time: 8 hours
Servings: 8

Ingredients:
- 4 cups low-sodium veggie stock
- 2 tablespoons Italian seasoning
- 1 pound sausage, no extra salt added and sliced
- A pinch of black pepper
- 2 pounds shrimp, deveined
- 2 tablespoons parsley, chopped
- 4 tablespoons olive oil

Directions:
In your slow cooker, mix stock with Italian seasoning, sausage, pepper, oil and shrimp, toss, cover, cook on Low for 8 hours, add parsley, toss, divide into small bowls and serve as an appetizer.
Enjoy!

Nutrition: calories 202, fat 3, fiber 5, carbs 14, protein 6

Salmon and Scallions Salad

Preparation time: 10 minutes
Cooking time: 2 hours
Servings: 4

Ingredients:

- 3 salmon fillets, skin on, boneless and cubed
- Zest of 1 lemon, grated
- 4 scallions, chopped
- 3 black peppercorns
- ½ teaspoon fennel seeds
- Black pepper to the taste
- 1 teaspoon white wine vinegar
- 2 cups low-sodium chicken stock
- ¼ cup dill, chopped

Directions:
In your slow cooker, mix lemon zest with scallions, peppercorns, fennel, pepper, vinegar, stock, dill and salmon, cover and cook on High for 2 hours. Divide salmon and scallions salad into bowls and serve warm as an appetizer.
Enjoy!

Nutrition: calories 202, fat 3, fiber 2, carbs 14, protein 11

Salmon Bites and Lemon Dressing

Preparation time: 10 minutes
Cooking time: 2 hours
Servings: 4

Ingredients:

- 4 salmon fillets, skinless, boneless and cubed
- 2 tablespoons chili pepper
- Juice of 1 lemon
- 1 lemon, sliced
- 1 cup low-sodium veggie stock
- 1 teaspoon sweet paprika
- 1 teaspoon basil, dried
- Salt and black pepper to the taste

Directions:
In your slow cooker, mix chili pepper with lemon juice, stock, paprika, basil, pepper and salmon, cover and cook on High for 2 hours. Divide salmon into bowls drizzle sauce from the pot all over and serve.
Enjoy!

Nutrition: calories 199, fat 4, fiber 7, carbs 14, protein 7

Dash Diet Slow Cooker Dessert Recipes

Easy Carrot and Pineapple Cake

Preparation time: 10 minutes
Cooking time: 2 hours and 30 minutes
Servings: 6

Ingredients:
- 1 cup pineapple, dried and chopped
- 4 carrots, chopped
- 1 and ½ cups whole wheat flour
- 1 cup dates, pitted and chopped
- ½ cup coconut flakes
- ½ teaspoon cinnamon powder
- Cooking spray

Directions:
Put carrots in your food processor and pulse. Add flour, dates, pineapple, coconut, cinnamon, and pulse very well again. Grease the slow cooker with the cooking spray, pour the cake mix, spread, cover and cook on High for 2 hours and 30 minutes. Leave the cake to cool down, slice and serve.
Enjoy!

Nutrition: calories 200, fat 2, fiber 4, carbs 16, protein 4

Coconut Green Tea Cream

Preparation time: 10 minutes
Cooking time: 1 hour
Servings: 4

Ingredients:
- 4 tablespoons low-fat coconut milk
- 1 cup fat-free coconut cream
- 3 tablespoons hot water
- 4 and ½ teaspoons green tea powder

Directions:
In a bowl, mix green tea powder with hot water, stir well and leave aside to cool down. In your slow cooker, mix the green tea with milk and cream, stir, cover, cook on High for 1 hour, transfer to a container and freeze before serving.
Enjoy!

Nutrition: calories 182, fat 2, fiber 5, carbs 12, protein 4

Sweet Coconut Figs

Preparation time: 6 minutes
Cooking time: 2 hours
Servings: 4

Ingredients:
- 2 tablespoons coconut butter, melted
- 12 figs, halved
- ¼ cup palm sugar
- 1 cup coconut cream

Directions:
In your slow cooker, mix the coconut butter with the figs, sugar and cream, stir, cover and cook on High for 2 hours. Divide into bowls and serve cold.
Enjoy!

Nutrition: calories 172, fat 2, fiber 1, carbs 8, protein 5

Chocolate and Vanilla Cream

Preparation time: 1 hour and 10 minutes
Cooking time: 2 hours
Servings: 4

Ingredients:
- 3 ounces dark and unsweetened chocolate
- 1 cup warm water
- 1 tablespoon vanilla extract
- 2 cups low-fat milk
- 3 tablespoons stevia
- 2 tablespoons gelatin

Directions:
In a bowl, mix warm water with gelatin, stir well and leave aside for 1 hour. Put this in your slow cooker, add milk, stevia, chocolate and vanilla, stir well, cover, cook on High for 2 hours, whisk the cream one more time, divide into bowls and serve.
Enjoy!

Nutrition: calories 210, fat 1, fiber 1, carbs 15, protein 6

Cinnamon Tomato Mix

Preparation time: 10 minutes
Cooking time: 4 hours
Servings: 4

Ingredients:
- 5 pounds tomatoes, blanched and peeled
- 3 cups coconut sugar
- 3 cups water, hot
- ½ teaspoon cinnamon powder
- 2 cinnamon sticks
- 2 teaspoons vanilla extract
- ½ teaspoon cloves, ground

Method:
In your slow cooker, mix the tomatoes with the water, cinnamon sticks, cinnamon powder, sugar, vanilla and cloves, stir, cover and cook on Low for 4 hours. Discard cinnamon sticks, leave the tomatoes aside to cool down, divide into bowls and serve!
Enjoy!

Nutrition: calories 210, fat 1, fiber 4, carbs 13, protein 4

Tomato Pie

Preparation time: 10 minutes
Cooking time: 3 hours
Servings: 6

Ingredients:
- 1 and ½ cups whole wheat flour
- 1 teaspoon cinnamon powder
- 1 teaspoon baking soda
- 1 teaspoon baking powder
- ¾ cup coconut sugar
- 1 cup tomatoes, blanched, peeled and chopped
- ½ cup olive oil
- 2 tablespoons apple cider vinegar
- Cooking spray

Directions:
In a bowl, mix flour with sugar, cinnamon, baking powder and soda and stir well. In another bowl, mix tomatoes with oil and cider vinegar and stir very well. Combine the 2 mixtures, stir, pour everything into your slow cooker greased with cooking spray, cover and cook on High for 3 hours. Leave the pie aside to cool down, slice and serve.
Enjoy!

Nutrition: calories 220, fat 8, fiber 7, carbs 11, protein 3

Berries and Orange Sauce

Preparation time: 10 minutes
Cooking time: 2 hours
Servings: 4

Ingredients:
- 1 cup orange juice
- 1 and ½ tablespoons stevia
- 1 and ½ tablespoons champagne vinegar
- 1 tablespoon olive oil
- 1 pound strawberries, halved
- 2 cups blueberries
- ¼ cup basil leaves, torn

Directions:
In your slow cooker, mix orange juice with sugar, vinegar, oil, blueberries and strawberries, toss to coat, cover, cook on High for 2 hours, divide into bowls, sprinkle basil on top and serve! Enjoy!

Nutrition: calories 199, fat 2, fiber 4, carbs 17, protein 5

Mango and Orange Sauce

Preparation time: 6 hours and 10 minutes
Cooking time: 2 hours
Servings: 3

Ingredients:
- 4 cups mango, peeled and cubed
- ¼ cup orange juice
- 6 tablespoons palm sugar
- 3 tablespoons lime juice

Directions:
Put mango, orange juice, lime juice and sugar, stir, cover and cook on High for 2 hours. Divide into bowls and keep in the fridge for 6 hours before serving.
Enjoy!

Nutrition: calories 120, fat 2, fiber 2, carbs 12, protein 3

Sweet Minty Grapefruit Mix

Preparation time: 10 minutes
Cooking time: 2 hours
Servings: 4

Ingredients:
- 1 cup water
- 2 cups grapefruit, peeled and cubed
- 1 cup palm sugar
- ½ cup mint, chopped
- 64 ounces red grapefruit juice

Directions:
In your slow cooker, mix the water with your grapefruit, sugar, mint and grapefruit juice, stir, cover and cook on High for 2 hours. Divide into bowls and serve cold.
Enjoy!

Nutrition: calories 130, fat 3, fiber 0, carbs 18, protein 3

Plums Stew

Preparation time: 10 minutes
Cooking time: 2 hours
Servings: 4

Ingredients:
- 16 ripe plums, stoned and halved
- 1 cup water
- ½ cup coconut sugar
- 5 cardamom pods, crushed

Directions:
In your slow cooker, mix the plums with the water, sugar and cardamom, stir, cover and cook on High for 2 hours. Divide into bowls and serve cold.
Enjoy!

Nutrition: calories 152, fat 3, fiber 2, carbs 15, protein 4

Cinnamon Apples

Preparation time: 10 minutes
Cooking time: 4 hours
Servings: 4

Ingredients:

- 4 big apples, cored and cut into wedges
- A handful raisins
- 1 tablespoon cinnamon powder
- 2 tablespoons natural apple juice
- 2 tablespoons honey

Directions:
In your slow cooker, mix the apples with the raisins, cinnamon, apple juice and honey, cover and cook on Low for 4 hours. Divide into bowls and serve warm.
Enjoy!

Nutrition: calories 182, fat 3, fiber 2, carbs 13, protein 3

Cocoa Cake

Preparation time: 10 minutes
Cooking time: 2 hours and 30 minutes
Servings: 8

Ingredients:

- 1 and ½ cup stevia
- 1 cup flour
- ¼ cup cocoa powder+ 2 tablespoons
- ½ cup chocolate almond milk
- 2 teaspoons baking powder
- 2 tablespoons canola oil
- 1 teaspoon vanilla extract
- 1 and ½ cups hot water
- Cooking spray

Directions:
In a bowl, mix flour with ¼-cup cocoa, baking powder, almond milk, oil and vanilla extract, whisk well and spread on the bottom of the slow cooker greased with cooking spray. In a separate bowl, mix stevia with the water and the rest of the cocoa, whisk well, spread over the batter, cover, and cook your cake on High for 2 hours and 30 minutes. Leave the cake to cool down, slice and serve.
Enjoy!

Nutrition: calories 200, fat 4, fiber 3, carbs 16, protein 4

Blueberry Pie

Preparation time: 10 minutes
Cooking time: 1 hour
Servings: 6

Ingredients:
- ½ cup whole wheat flour
- ¼ teaspoon baking powder
- ¼ teaspoon stevia
- ¼ cup blueberries
- 1/3 cup almond milk
- 1 teaspoon olive oil
- ½ teaspoon lemon zest, grated
- 1 teaspoon vanilla extract
- Cooking spray

Directions:
In a bowl, mix flour with baking powder, stevia, blueberries, milk, oil, lemon zest and vanilla extract, whisk, pour into your slow cooker lined with parchment paper and greased with the cooking spray, cover and cook on High for 1 hour. Leave the pie to cool down, slice and serve. Enjoy!

Nutrition: calories 200, fat 4, fiber 4, carbs 10, protein 4

Coconut Peach Cobbler

Preparation time: 10 minutes
Cooking time: 4 hours
Servings: 4

Ingredients:
- 4 cups peaches, peeled and sliced
- ¼ cup coconut sugar
- ½ teaspoon cinnamon powder
- 1 and ½ cups whole wheat sweet crackers, crushed
- ¼ cup stevia
- 1 teaspoon vanilla extract
- ¼ teaspoon nutmeg, ground
- ½ cup almond milk
- Cooking spray

Directions:
In a bowl, mix peaches with sugar, cinnamon, and stir. In a separate bowl, mix crackers with stevia, nutmeg, almond milk and vanilla extract and stir. Spray your slow cooker with cooking spray, spread peaches on the bottom, and add the crackers mix, spread, cover and cook on Low for 4 hours. Divide into bowls and serve.
Enjoy!

Nutrition: calories 212, fat 4, fiber 4, carbs 14, protein 4

Poached Strawberries

Preparation time: 10 minutes
Cooking time: 3 hours
Servings: 10

Ingredients:
- 2 tablespoons lemon juice
- 1 cup water
- 2 pounds strawberries
- 4 cups coconut sugar
- 1 teaspoon cinnamon powder
- 1 teaspoon vanilla extract

Directions:
In your slow cooker, mix strawberries with water, coconut sugar, lemon juice, cinnamon and vanilla, stir, cover, cook on Low for 3 hours, divide into bowls and serve cold.
Enjoy!

Nutrition: calories 211, fat 3, fiber 1, carbs 13, protein 4

Poached Bananas

Preparation time: 10 minutes
Cooking time: 2 hours
Servings: 4

Ingredients:
- Juice of ½ lemon
- 3 tablespoons agave nectar
- 1 tablespoon coconut oil
- 4 bananas, peeled and sliced
- ½ teaspoon cardamom seeds

Directions:
Arrange bananas in your slow cooker, add agave nectar, lemon juice, oil and cardamom, cover, cook on Low for 2 hours, divide everything into bowls and serve with.
Enjoy!

Nutrition: calories 200, fat 1, fiber 2, carbs 14, protein 3

Orange and Pecans Cake

Preparation time: 10 minutes
Cooking time: 5 hours
Servings: 4

Ingredients:
- Cooking spray
- 1 teaspoon baking powder
- 1 cup almond flour
- 1 cup coconut sugar
- ½ teaspoon cinnamon powder
- 3 tablespoons coconut oil, melted
- ½ cup almond milk
- ½ cup pecans, chopped
- ¾ cup water
- ½ cup orange peel, grated
- 1 cup orange juice

Directions:
In a bowl, mix flour with half of the sugar, baking powder, cinnamon, 2 tablespoons oil, milk and pecans, stir and pour this in your slow cooker greased with cooking spray. Heat up a small pan over medium heat, add water, orange juice, orange peel, the rest of the oil and the rest of the sugar, stir, bring to a boil, pour over the mix in the slow cooker, cover and cook on Low for 5 hours. Divide into bowls and serve cold.
Enjoy!

Nutrition: calories 202, fat 3, fiber 6, carbs 14, protein 4

Poached Pears

Preparation time: 10 minutes
Cooking time: 4 hours
Servings: 4

Ingredients:
- 4 pears, peeled and cored
- 2 cups grapefruit juice
- ¼ cup maple syrup
- 2 teaspoons cinnamon powder
- 1 tablespoon ginger, grated

Directions:
In your slow cooker, mix pears with grapefruit juice, maple syrup, cinnamon and ginger, cover, cook on Low for 4 hours, divide everything into bowls and serve.
Enjoy!

Nutrition: calories 200, fat 4, fiber 2, carbs 13, protein 4

Pumpkin Pie

Preparation time: 10 minutes
Cooking time: 2 hours
Servings: 10

Ingredients:
- 1 and ½ teaspoons baking powder
- Cooking spray
- 1 cup pumpkin puree
- 2 cups almond flour
- ½ teaspoon baking soda
- 1 and ½ teaspoons cinnamon powder
- ¼ teaspoon ginger, ground
- 1 tablespoon coconut oil, melted
- 1 egg, whisked
- 1 tablespoon vanilla extract
- 1/3 cup maple syrup
- 1 teaspoon lemon juice

Directions:
In a bowl, flour with baking powder, baking soda, cinnamon, ginger, egg, oil, vanilla, pumpkin puree, maple syrup and lemon juice, stir and pour in your slow cooker greased with cooking spray and lined with parchment paper, cover the pot and cook on Low for 2 hours and 20 minutes. Leave the pie to cool down, slice and serve.
Enjoy!

Nutrition: calories 211, fat 5, fiber 2, carbs 16, protein 7

Lemon Cream

Preparation time: 10 minutes
Cooking time: 3 hours
Servings: 10

Ingredients:
- 2 pounds lemons, washed, peeled and sliced
- 2 pounds coconut sugar
- 1 tablespoon vinegar

Directions:
In your slow cooker, mix lemons with coconut sugar and vinegar, stir, cover, cook on High for 3 hours, blend using an immersion blender, divide into small bowls and serve.
Enjoy!

Nutrition: calories 151, fat 3, fiber 5, carbs 17, protein 4

Minty Rhubarb Dip

Preparation time: 10 minutes
Cooking time: 3 hours
Servings: 8

Ingredients:
- 1/3 cup water
- 4 pounds rhubarb, chopped
- 1 cup coconut sugar
- 1 tablespoon mint, chopped

Directions:
In your slow cooker, mix water with rhubarb, sugar and mint, stir, cover, cook on High for 3 hours, blend using an immersion blender, divide into cups and serve cold.
Enjoy!

Nutrition: calories 170, fat 1, fiber 4, carbs 13, protein 4

Cherry Jam

Preparation time: 10 minutes
Cooking time: 3 hours
Servings: 6

Ingredients:
- 2 tablespoons lemon juice
- 3 tablespoons gelatin
- 4 cups cherries, pitted
- 2 cups coconut sugar

Directions:
In your slow cooker, mix lemon juice with gelatin, cherries and coconut sugar, stir, cover, cook on High for 3 hours, divide into bowls and serve cold.
Enjoy!

Nutrition: calories 200, fat 3, fiber 1, carbs 14, protein 3

Cinnamon Rice Pudding

Preparation time: 10 minutes
Cooking time: 5 hours
Servings: 4

Ingredients:
- 6 and ½ cups water
- 1 cup coconut sugar
- 2 cups white rice
- 2 cinnamon sticks
- ½ cup coconut, shredded

Directions:
In your slow cooker, mix water with the rice, sugar, cinnamon and coconut, stir, cover, cook on High for 5 hours, discard cinnamon, divide pudding into bowls and serve warm.
Enjoy!

Nutrition: calories 173, fat 4, fiber 6, carbs 9, protein 4

Almond Chocolate Bars

Preparation time: 10 minutes
Cooking time: 2 hours and 30 minutes
Servings: 12

Ingredients:
- 1 egg white
- ¼ cup coconut oil, melted
- 1 cup coconut sugar
- ½ teaspoon vanilla extract
- 1 teaspoon baking powder
- 1 and ½ cups almond meal
- ½ cup dark chocolate chips

Directions:
In a bowl, mix the oil with sugar, vanilla extract, egg white, baking powder and almond flour and whisk well. Fold in chocolate chips and stir gently. Line your slow cooker with parchment paper, grease it, add cookie mix, press on the bottom, cover and cook on low for 2 hours and 30 minutes. Take cookie sheet out of the slow cooker, cut into medium bars and serve.
Enjoy!

Nutrition: calories 200, fat 2, fiber 1, carbs 13, protein 6

Pineapple Pudding

Preparation time: 10 minutes
Cooking time: 5 hours
Servings: 4

Ingredients:
- Cooking spray
- 1 teaspoon baking powder
- 1 cup coconut flour
- 3 tablespoons stevia
- 3 tablespoons avocado oil
- ½ cup coconut milk
- ½ cup pecans, chopped
- ½ cup pineapple, chopped
- ½ cup lemon zest, grated
- 1 cup pineapple juice, natural

Directions:
Spray your slow cooker with cooking spray. In a bowl, mix flour with stevia, baking powder, oil, milk, pecans, pineapple, lemon zest and pineapple juice, stir well, pour into your slow cooker greased with cooking spray, cover and cook on Low for 5 hours. Divide into bowls and serve. Enjoy!

Nutrition: calories 172, fat 3, fiber 1, carbs 14, protein 5

Delicious Apple Mix

Preparation time: 10 minutes
Cooking time: 4 hours
Servings: 4

Ingredients:
- Cooking spray
- 2 teaspoons lemon juice
- 3 tablespoons stevia
- ¼ teaspoon ginger, grated
- 6 big apples, roughly chopped
- ½ cup almond flour
- ¼ teaspoon cinnamon powder
- ¼ cup coconut oil, melted
- ½ cup walnuts, chopped

Directions:
Spray your slow cooker with cooking spray. In a bowl, mix stevia with lemon juice, ginger, apples and cinnamon, stir and pour into your slow cooker. In another bowl, mix flour with walnuts and oil, stir, pour into the slow cooker, cover, and cook on Low for 4 hours. Divide into bowls and serve.
Enjoy!

Nutrition: calories 200, fat 3, fiber 2, carbs 7, protein 5

Avocado Pudding

Preparation time: 6 minutes
Cooking time: 1 hour
Servings: 4

Ingredients:
- ½ cup coconut water
- 1 and ½ cup avocado, pitted, peeled and chopped
- 2 tablespoons green tea powder
- 2 teaspoons lime zest, grated
- 1 tablespoon stevia

Directions:
In your slow cooker, mix coconut water with avocado, green tea powder, lime zest and stevia, stir, cover, cook on Low for 1 hour, divide into bowls and serve.
Enjoy!

Nutrition: calories 207, fat 4, fiber 8, carbs 17, protein 7

Chia Pudding

Preparation time: 10 minutes
Cooking time: 1 hour
Servings: 4

Ingredients:
- 1 and ½ cup coconut milk
- ½ cup pumpkin puree
- 2 tablespoons maple syrup
- ½ cup chia seeds
- ½ teaspoon cinnamon powder
- ¼ teaspoon ginger, grated

Directions:
In your slow cooker, mix the milk with the pumpkin puree, maple syrup, chia, cinnamon and ginger, stir, cover, cook on High for 1 hour, divide into bowls and serve.
Enjoy!

Nutrition: calories 145, fat 2, fiber 7, carbs 14, protein 4

Grapefruit Compote

Preparation time: 10 minutes
Cooking time: 2 hours
Servings: 6

Ingredients:
- 1 cup water
- 1 cup honey
- ½ cup mint, chopped
- 64 ounces red grapefruit juice
- 2 grapefruits, peeled and chopped

Directions:
In your slow cooker, mix grapefruit with water, honey, mint and grapefruit juice, stir, cover, cook on High for 2 hours, divide into bowls and serve cold.
Enjoy!

Nutrition: calories 140, fat 1, fiber, 2, carbs 14, protein 4

Dark Cherry and Cocoa Compote

Preparation time: 10 minutes
Cooking time: 2 hours
Servings: 6

Ingredients:
- ½ cup dark cocoa powder
- ¾ cup red grape juice
- ¼ cup maple syrup
- 1 pound dark cherries, pitted and halved
- 2 tablespoons stevia
- 2 cups water

Directions:
In your slow cooker, mix cocoa powder with grape juice, maple syrup, cherries, water and stevia, stir, cover, cook on High for 2 hours, divide into bowls and serve cold.
Enjoy!

Nutrition: calories 200, fat 1, fiber 4, carbs 14, protein 4

Citrus Apples and Pears Mix

Preparation time: 10 minutes
Cooking time: 1 hour
Servings: 6

Ingredients:
- 1 quart water
- 2 tablespoons stevia
- ½ pound apple, cored and cut into wedges
- ½ pound pears, cored and cut into wedges
- 5 star anise
- 2 cinnamon sticks
- Zest of 1 orange, grated
- Zest of 1 lemon, grated

Directions:
Put the water, stevia, apples, pears, star anise, and cinnamon, orange and lemon zest in your slow cooker, cover, cook on High for 1 hour, divide into bowls and serve cold.
Enjoy!

Nutrition: calories 128, fat 3, fiber 2, carbs 6, protein 2

Pears Cake

Preparation time: 10 minutes
Cooking time: 2 hours and 30 minutes
Servings: 6

Ingredients:
- 3 cups pears, cored and cubed
- 3 tablespoons stevia
- 1 tablespoon vanilla extract
- 2 eggs
- 1 tablespoon pumpkin pie spice
- 2 cups coconut flour
- 1 tablespoon baking powder
- 1 tablespoon avocado oil

Directions:
In a bowl mix eggs with the oil, spice, vanilla, pears and stevia and whisk well. In another bowl, mix baking powder with flour, stir, add to apples mix, stir again, transfer to your slow cooker, cover, cook on High for 2 hours and 30 minutes, slice and serve cold.
Enjoy!

Nutrition: calories 200, fat 2, fiber 2, carbs 12, protein 4

Cocoa Pudding

Preparation time: 10 minutes
Cooking time: 1 hour
Servings: 2

Ingredients:
- 2 tablespoons water
- 2 tablespoon gelatin
- 4 tablespoons stevia
- 4 tablespoons cocoa powder
- 2 cups coconut milk, hot

Directions:
In a bowl, mix milk with stevia and cocoa powder and stir well. Add the gelatin mixed with water, stir well, add to your slow cooker, cook on High for 1 hour, divide into bowls and serve cold.
Enjoy!

Nutrition: calories 180, fat 2, fiber 1, carbs 13, protein 3

Raspberry Energy Bars

Preparation time: 10 minutes
Cooking time: 1 hour
Servings: 12

Ingredients:
- ½ cup low-fat butter
- ½ cup coconut oil, melted
- ½ cup coconut, unsweetened and shredded
- 1 cup raspberries
- 3 tablespoons stevia

Directions:
In your slow cooker, mix the butter with the oil, coconut, raspberries and stevia, toss, cover and cook on High for 1 hour. Spread on a lined baking sheet, keep in the fridge for a few hours, cut into bars and serve.
Enjoy!

Nutrition: calories 174, fat 5, fiber 2, carbs 4, protein 7

Berries Cream

Preparation time: 10 minutes
Cooking time: 1 hour
Servings: 10

Ingredients:
- 8 ounces mascarpone cheese
- 1 teaspoon stevia
- 1 cup coconut cream
- 1 pint blueberries

Directions:
In your slow cooker, mix the cream with stevia, mascarpone and the blueberries, stir, cover, cook on Low for 1 hour, divide bowls and serve cold.
Enjoy!

Nutrition: calories 183, fat 4, fiber 1, carbs 10, protein 4

Blackberries and Cocoa Pudding

Preparation time: 10 minutes
Cooking time: 1 hour
Servings: 4

Ingredients:
- 3 tablespoons cocoa powder
- 14 ounces coconut cream
- 2 cups blackberries
- 2 tablespoons stevia

Directions:
In your slow cooker, mix the cream with cocoa, stevia and blackberries, stir, cover, cook on High for 1 hour, divide into dessert cups and serve cold.
Enjoy!

Nutrition: calories 145, fat 4, fiber 2, carbs 6, protein 2

Peach Compote

Preparation time: 10 minutes
Cooking time: 1 hour and 30 minutes
Servings: 6

Ingredients:
- 4 tablespoons palm sugar
- 4 cups peaches, cored and roughly chopped
- 6 tablespoons natural apple juice
- 2 teaspoons lemon zest, grated

Directions:
In your slow cooker, mix peaches with sugar, apple juice and lemon zest, stir, cover, cook on High for 1 hour and 30 minutes, divide into bowls and serve cold.
Enjoy!

Nutrition: calories 182, fat 2, fiber 2, carbs 8, protein 5

Zucchini Cake

Preparation time: 10 minutes
Cooking time: 4 hours
Servings: 6

Ingredients:
- 1 cup natural applesauce
- 3 eggs, whisked
- 1 tablespoon vanilla extract
- 4 tablespoons stevia
- 2 cups zucchini, grated
- 2 and ½ cups coconut flour
- ½ cup baking cocoa powder
- 1 teaspoon baking soda
- ¼ teaspoon baking powder
- 1 teaspoon cinnamon powder
- Cooking spray

Directions:
Grease your slow with cooking spray, add zucchini, sugar, vanilla, eggs, applesauce, flour, cocoa powder, baking soda, baking powder and cinnamon, whisk, cook on High for 4 hours, cool down, slice and serve.
Enjoy!

Nutrition: calories 171, fat 4, fiber 6, carbs 10, protein 3

Grapes Pudding

Preparation time: 5 minutes
Cooking time: 1 hour
Servings: 4

Ingredients:
- 2 cups grapes, halved
- 2 cups coconut milk
- 1 tablespoon coconut oil
- 3 tablespoons stevia
- ½ teaspoon cinnamon powder
- 1 cup coconut flakes
- ½ cup walnuts, chopped

Directions:
In your slow cooker, combine the milk with stevia, oil, coconut, cinnamon, grapes and walnuts, stir, cover, cook on High for 1 hour, divide into bowls and serve cold.
Enjoy!

Nutrition: calories 182, fat 3, fiber 4, carbs 10, protein 7

Apricot Cream

Preparation time: 10 minutes
Cooking time: 3 hours
Servings: 10

Ingredients:
- 2 tablespoons lemon juice
- 2 pounds apricots, chopped
- 4 cups coconut sugar
- 1 teaspoon cinnamon powder
- 1 teaspoon vanilla extract

Directions:
In your slow cooker, mix the apricots with the sugar, lemon juice, cinnamon and vanilla, cover, cook on Low for 3 hours, blend using an immersion blender, divide into bowls and serve cold.
Enjoy!

Nutrition: calories 140, fat 0, fiber 1, carbs 11, protein 3

Poached Apples

Preparation time: 10 minutes
Cooking time: 4 hours
Servings: 6

Ingredients:
- 6 apples, cored, peeled and sliced
- 1 cup apple juice, natural
- Cooking spray
- 1 cup coconut sugar
- 1 tablespoon cinnamon powder

Directions:
Grease your slow cooker with cooking spray, add apples, juice, sugar and cinnamon, stir, cover, cook on High for 4 hours, divide into bowls and serve cold.
Enjoy!

Nutrition: calories 180, fat 5, fiber 5, carbs 8, protein 4

Stewed Cardamom Pears

Preparation time: 10 minutes
Cooking time: 4 hours
Servings: 4

Ingredients:
- 4 pears, peeled and tops cut off and cored
- 5 cardamom pods
- 2 cups apple juice
- ¼ cup maple syrup
- 1-inch ginger, grated

Directions:
Put the pears in your slow cooker, add cardamom, apple juice, maple syrup and ginger, cover, cook on Low for 4 hours, divide into bowls and serve.
Enjoy!

Nutrition: calories 172, fat 4, fiber 2, carbs 12, protein 4

Maple Grapes Compote

Preparation time: 10 minutes
Cooking time: 4 hours
Servings: 2

Ingredients:
- 1 cup water
- 1 cup maple syrup
- 12 ounces red grape juice
- 2 cups green grapes, halved

Directions:
In your slow cooker, mix grapes with water, maple syrup and grape juice, stir, cover, cook on Low for 4 hours, divide into bowls and serve cold.
Enjoy!

Nutrition: calories 161, fat 1, fiber, 2, carbs 8, protein 1

Brown Rice Pudding

Preparation time: 10 minutes
Cooking time: 4 hours
Servings: 6

Ingredients:
- 14 ounces low-fat coconut milk
- 1 and 2/3 cups low-fat milk
- ¼ cup honey
- 1 teaspoon vanilla extract
- ½ cup raisins
- 1 teaspoon cinnamon powder
- 2/3 cup brown rice

Directions:
In your slow cooker, mix the coconut milk with the low-fat milk, honey, vanilla, cinnamon and raisins and whisk well. Add the rice, stir, cover and cook on Low for 4 hours. Divide into bowls and serve warm.
Enjoy!

Nutrition: calories 234, fat 12, fiber 1, carbs 20, protein 4

Berry Cobbler

Preparation time: 10 minutes
Cooking time: 2 hours and 30 minutes
Servings: 8

Ingredients:
- 1 and ¼ cups almond flour
- 1 cup coconut sugar
- 1 teaspoon baking powder
- ½ teaspoon cinnamon powder
- 1 egg
- ¼ cup low-fat milk
- 2 tablespoons olive oil
- 2 cups raspberries
- 2 cups blueberries
- Cooking spray

Directions:
In a bowl, mix the almond flour with the sugar, baking powder and cinnamon and stir. In another bowl, mix the egg with the milk, oil, raspberries and blueberries and stir. Combine the 2 mixtures, pour everything into your slow cooker greased with the cooking spray, cover and cook on High for 2 hours and 30 minutes. Divide into bowls and serve.
Enjoy!

Nutrition: calories 250, fat 4, fiber 4, carbs 30, protein 3

Pumpkin Apple Dip

Preparation time: 10 minutes
Cooking time: 8 hours
Servings: 8

Ingredients:
- 8 apples, cored, peeled and sliced
- 1 cup pumpkin puree
- 1/3 cup palm sugar
- 1/3 cup water
- ½ teaspoon pumpkin pie spice
- ¼ teaspoon nutmeg, ground

Directions:
In your slow cooker, combine the apples with the sugar, pumpkin puree, water, spice and nutmeg, stir, cover and cook on Low for 8 hours. Blend using an immersion blender, divide into bowls and serve as a sweet dip.
Enjoy!

Nutrition: calories 100, fat 1, fiber 5, carbs 20, protein 4

Apple Dip

Preparation time: 10 minutes
Cooking time: 3 hours
Servings: 4

Ingredients:
- 8 apples, cored and chopped
- 2 drops cinnamon oil
- 1 cup water
- 1 teaspoon cinnamon powder

Directions:
Put apples in your slow cooker, add the water, oil and cinnamon, cover, cook on High for 3 hours, blend using an immersion blender, divide into bowls and serve cold.
Enjoy!

Nutrition: calories 121, fat 2, fiber 6, carbs 17, protein 4

Cranberry Dip

Preparation time: 10 minutes
Cooking time: 2 hours and 30 minutes
Servings: 4

Ingredients:
- 2 and ½ teaspoons orange zest, grated
- 12 ounces cranberries
- ¼ cup orange juice
- 2 tablespoons maple syrup
- 1 cup coconut sugar

Directions:
In your slow cooker, mix orange juice with maple syrup, orange zest, sugar and cranberries, stir, cover and cook on High for 2 hours and 30 minutes. Blend using an immersion blender, divide into bowls and serve.
Enjoy!

Nutrition: calories 162, fat 4, fiber 8, carbs 18, protein 6

Sweet Mango Dip

Preparation time: 10 minutes
Cooking time: 3 hours
Servings: 4

Ingredients:
- 1 tablespoon avocado oil
- ¼ teaspoon cardamom powder
- 2 tablespoons ginger, grated
- ½ teaspoon cinnamon
- 4 mangos, cored and chopped
- 1 apple, cored and chopped
- ¼ cup raisins
- 1 and ¼ cup coconut sugar
- 1 and ¼ apple cider vinegar

Directions:
In your slow cooker, mix the oil with cardamom, ginger, cinnamon, mangos, apple, raisins, sugar and cider, stir, cover and cook on High for 3 hours. Blend using an immersion blender, divide into bowls and serve.
Enjoy!

Nutrition: calories 121, fat 4, fiber 7, carbs 15, protein 3

Plum Dip

Preparation time: 10 minutes
Cooking time: 3 hours
Servings: 20

Ingredients:
- 3 pounds plums, pitted and chopped
- 2 apples, cored and chopped
- 4 tablespoons ginger, ground
- 4 tablespoons cinnamon powder
- 4 tablespoons allspice, ground
- ¾ pound coconut sugar

Directions:
Put plums and apples in your slow cooker, add ginger, cinnamon, allspice and sugar, stir, cover and cook on High for 3 hours. Pulse using an immersion blender, divide into bowls and serve.
Enjoy!

Nutrition: calories 152, fat 3, fiber 8, carbs 18, protein 12

Conclusion

The Dash diet is one of the healthiest ever! It's a lifestyle you need to adopt in order to lower your blood pressure. The Dash diet will change your life forever and it will transform you into a healthy and happy person.

As you now know, this diet is not a restrictive one. You need to cut down your fat and sodium intakes and to increase your veggie, legumes, beans, whole grains and fruits servings!

You have discovered so many amazing Dash diet recipes in this magnificent cooking journal but the best thing about them is that they are all made in one of the most popular kitchen tools ever: in a slow cooker!

This is so amazing, isn't it?

Then what are you waiting for? Get your hands on a copy of this amazing cookbook and see what this Dash diet is all about!

Enjoy!

Recipe Index

A

Acorn Squash Mix, 78
Almond and Cherries Oats, 25
Almond Chocolate Bars, 122
Apple and Raisins Oatmeal, 18
Apple Brussels Sprouts, 76
Apple Dip, 134
Apples and Dates Oatmeal, 21
Apples and Sauce, 31
Apricot Cream, 130
Artichoke and Beans Spread, 86
Artichoke and Spinach Dip, 95
Artichokes Mix, 69
Asian Green Beans, 80
Asian Salmon, 47
Asparagus Mix, 70
Asparagus Snack, 89
Avocado Pudding, 124

B

Baby Spinach and Avocado Mix, 83
Basil and Oregano Mushrooms, 84
Beet and Celery Spread, 104
Beet Soup, 42
Berries and Orange Sauce, 114
Berries Cream, 128
Berry Cobbler, 133
Black Bean and Corn Mix, 70
Black Bean Salsa, 94
Black Beans and Mango Mix, 46
Blackberries and Cocoa Pudding, 128
Black-Eyed Peas Mix, 65
Blueberry Pie, 117
Breakfast Berries Compote, 20
Breakfast Nuts and Squash Bowls, 29
Breakfast Potatoes, 29
Breakfast Veggie Omelet, 17
Broccoli and Cauliflower Soup, 43
Broccoli Mix, 61
Brown Rice Pudding, 132
Bulgur and Beans Salad, 96
Butternut Mix, 64
Butternut Squash Cream, 44

C

Cabbage, Radish and Carrot Mix, 85
Cajun Peas Spread, 92
Carrot and Zucchini Oatmeal, 11
Cashew Spread, 93
Cauliflower Rice and Mushrooms, 80
Celery Mix, 71
Cherry Jam, 121
Chia Pudding, 28
Chia Pudding, 124
Chicken and Rice Soup, 41
Chicken and Veggies, 38

Chicken Breast and Cinnamon Veggie Mix, 53
Chicken Breast Stew, 52
Chicken Omelet, 35
Chicken Tacos, 36
Chickpeas Hummus, 88
Chickpeas Mix, 44
Chickpeas Side Dish, 75
Chili Cauliflower Dip, 106
Chili Coconut Corn Spread, 94
Chocolate and Vanilla Cream, 112
Cinnamon Apples, 116
Cinnamon Rice Pudding, 122
Cinnamon Tomato Mix, 113
Citrus Apples and Pears Mix, 126
Citrus Turkey Mix, 60
Clams Salad, 105
Classic Peas and Carrots, 63
Cocoa Cake, 116
Cocoa Pudding, 127
Coconut Broccoli, 79
Coconut Clams, 49
Coconut Green Tea Cream, 111
Coconut Peach Cobbler, 117
Coconut Quinoa Mix, 11
Coconut Salmon Soup, 57
Coconut Spinach Dip, 93
Cod Salsa, 108
Corn Pudding, 24
Corn Salad, 72
Cranberries, Apple and Onion Salad, 106
Cranberries, Cauliflower and Mushroom Mix, 81
Cranberry Dip, 134
Cranberry Toast, 25
Creamy and Cheesy Spinach, 82
Creamy Cauliflower Rice, 81
Creamy Corn, 62
Creamy Endive Salad, 105
Creamy Fish Curry, 58
Creamy Mushrooms Mix, 68
Creamy Seafood and Veggies Soup, 50
Creamy Veggie Omelet, 34

D

Dark Cherry and Cocoa Compote, 125
Delicious Apple Granola Breakfast, 10
Delicious Apple Mix, 123
Delicious Banana and Coconut Oatmeal, 10
Delicious Black Bean Chili, 37
Delicious Black Bean Soup, 41
Delicious Frittata, 16
Delicious Omelet, 19
Delicious Peanut Butter Oats, 18
Delicious Tomato Cream, 42
Delicious Veggie Soup, 40
Dill Cauliflower Mash, 82

Dill Walnuts and Seeds Mix, 101
Easy Breakfast Casserole, 13
Easy Burrito Bowls, 26
Easy Cabbage, 78
Easy Carrot and Pineapple Cake, 111
Easy Carrot Oatmeal, 27
Easy Green Beans, 62
Easy Navy Beans Soup, 46
Easy Pork Party Meatballs, 98
Easy Potatoes Mix, 65
Easy Pulled Chicken, 39
Easy Pumpkin Oatmeal, 15
Easy Quinoa and Oats, 14
Easy Zucchini Rolls, 103
Egg Casserole, 30
Eggplant Salsa, 86

F
Fruits and Cereals Mix, 20

G
Garlic and Rosemary Potato Mix, 76
Garlicky Potato Mash, 74
Ginger Beets, 69
Grapefruit Compote, 125
Grapes Pudding, 130
Greek Cod Mix, 58
Greek Dash Casserole, 12
Greek Pork, 55
Green Beans and Corn Mix, 66
Ground Pork and Veggies Soup, 57

H
Herbed Salmon, 49
Hot Mackerel, 59

I
Italian Beans Mix, 77
Italian Chicken, 53
Italian Nuts Mix, 101
Italian Shrimp Salad, 109
Italian Tomato Appetizer, 87
Italian Veggie Dip, 92
Italian Zucchini and Squash, 79

J
Jumbo Shrimp Appetizer, 103
K
Kale Side Dish, 71

L
Leeks, Kale and Sweet Potato Mix, 30
Lemon and Spinach Trout, 51
Lemon Cream, 120

M
Mango and Orange Sauce, 114
Maple Apples, 31
Maple Grapes Compote, 132
Maple Pork Tenderloin, 54
Mediterranean Chicken, 40

Mexican Casserole, 22
Mexican Chicken, 51
Mexican Dash Diet Eggs, 13
Mexican Pork Mix, 54
Minty Okra, 84
Minty Rhubarb Dip, 121
Minty Spinach Dip, 91
Mushroom and Bell Pepper Dip, 95
Mushroom Mix, 67
Mushroom Pilaf, 63
Mussels Mix, 59

N
Navy Beans Stew, 45

O
Orange and Pecans Cake, 119
Orange and Strawberry Breakfast Mix, 19

P
Peach Compote, 129
Pears Cake, 126
Pepper and Chickpeas Dip, 90
Pineapple and Carrot Mix, 33
Pineapple Chicken Wings, 97
Pineapple Pudding, 123
Plum Dip, 135
Plums Stew, 115
Poached Apples, 131
Poached Bananas, 118
Poached Pears, 119
Poached Strawberries, 118
Pork and Cabbage Stew, 55
Pork Roast Soup, 56
Pork Rolls, 98
Potatoes Stew, 45
Pumpkin Apple Dip, 133
Pumpkin Butter, 32
Pumpkin Pie, 120

Q
Quinoa Casserole, 36
Quinoa Curry, 37

R
Raspberry Energy Bars, 127
Raspberry Oatmeal, 15
Rich Lentils Soup, 43
Roast and Veggies, 56

S
Sage Sweet Potatoes, 74
Salmon and Carrots Appetizer Salad, 109
Salmon and Scallions Salad, 110
Salmon Appetizer Salad, 104
Salmon Bites and Lemon Dressing, 110
Salmon Omelet, 34
Sausage Meatballs and Apricot Sauce, 107
Sausage Side Dish, 64
Scrambled Eggs, 17
Scrambled Eggs and Veggies, 21

Seafood Gumbo, 50
Seafood Stew, 48
Shrimp and Beans Appetizer Salad, 89
Shrimp Cocktail, 108
Shrimp Frittata, 22
Simple Apple Oatmeal, 14
Simple Banana Bread, 12
Simple Blueberries Oatmeal, 27
Simple Parsnips Mix, 83
Simple Swiss Chard Mix, 85
Slow Cooked Tuna, 48
Spiced Cabbage, 73
Spiced Carrots, 66
Spiced Coconut Oats, 26
Spiced Pecans Snack, 97
Spicy Eggplant, 72
Spinach and Beans Mix, 73
Spinach and Rice, 68
Spinach Frittata, 16
Spinach Pie, 33
Spinach Soup, 47
Squash and Apples Breakfast Mix, 23
Squash and Grains Mix, 67
Sriracha Chicken Dip, 107
Stewed Cardamom Pears, 131
Stuffed Chicken, 100
Stuffed White Mushrooms, 87
Succulent Pork Roast, 38

Sweet Coconut Figs, 112
Sweet Mango Dip, 135
Sweet Minty Grapefruit Mix, 115
Sweet Pineapple Snack, 88
Sweet Potato and Sausage Pie, 32
Sweet Potatoes Mix, 24

T
Tasty Bean Side Dish, 61
Tofu and Veggies Frittata, 28
Tofu Scramble, 23
Tomato Dip, 102
Tomato Pie, 113
Tomato Salsa, 99
Tomato Shrimp Salad, 100
Tomatoes, Okra and Zucchini Mix, 77
Turkey Breast and Sweet Potato Mix, 52
Turkey Chili, 39
Turkey Wings and Veggies, 60
Turnips and Cauliflower Spread, 91

W
Warm Eggplant Salad, 75
Warm French Veggie Salad, 96
White Bean Spread, 90
White Fish Sticks, 99

Z
Zucchini Cake, 129
Zucchini Dip, 102

Copyright 2018 by Marta Getty All rights reserved.

All rights Reserved. No part of this publication or the information in it may be quoted from or reproduced in any form by means such as printing, scanning, photocopying or otherwise without prior written permission of the copyright holder.

Disclaimer and Terms of Use: Effort has been made to ensure that the information in this book is accurate and complete, however, the author and the publisher do not warrant the accuracy of the information, text and graphics contained within the book due to the rapidly changing nature of science, research, known and unknown facts and internet. The Author and the publisher do not hold any responsibility for errors, omissions or contrary interpretation of the subject matter herein. This book is presented solely for motivational and informational purposes only.

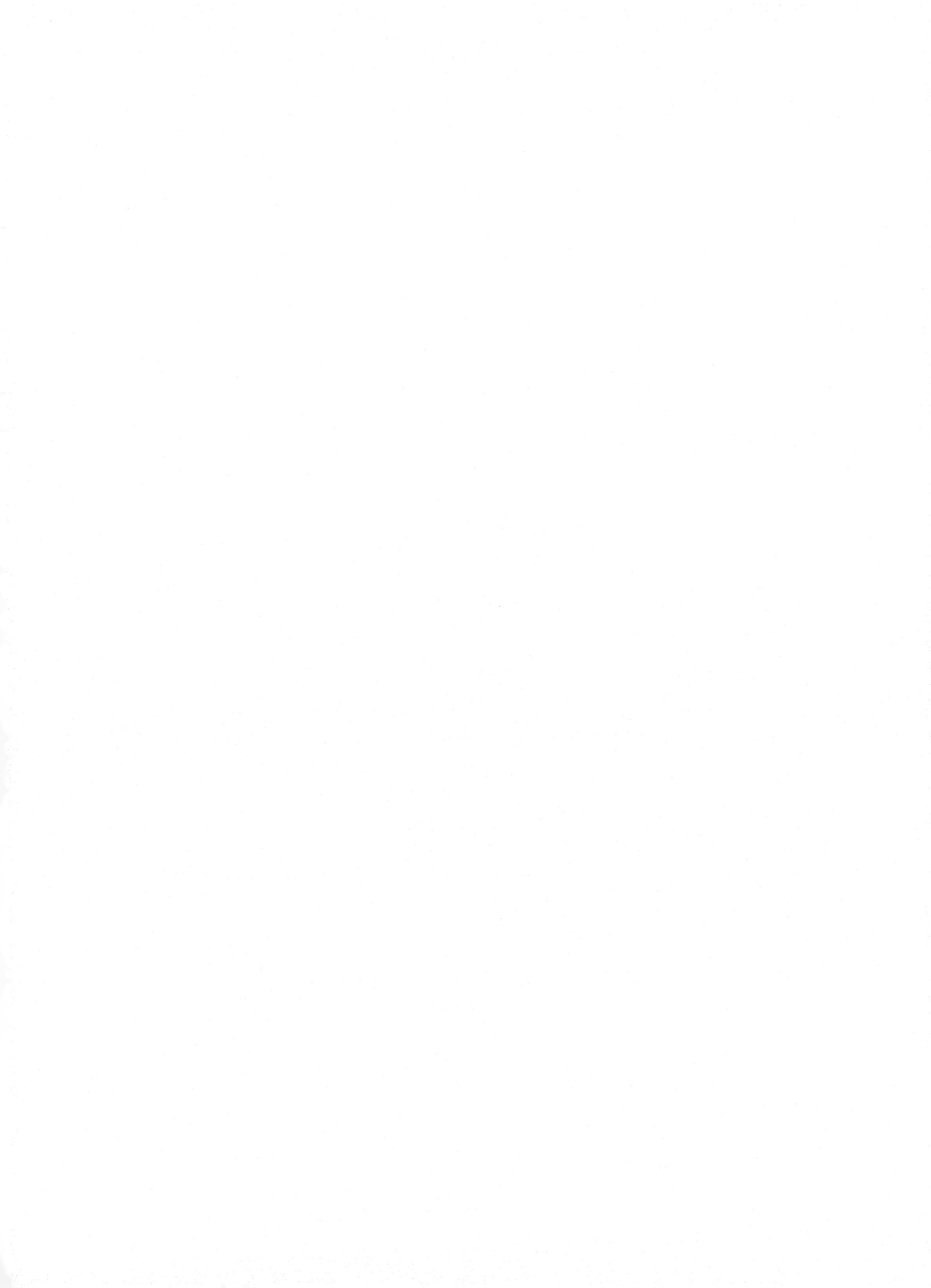

CPSIA information can be obtained
at www.ICGtesting.com
Printed in the USA
BVOW09s1127010418
512173BV00018B/366/P